MED-MAL

J. Annie

MED-MAL

Copyright © 2019

All rights reserved. No part of this book may be reproduced or by any means without prior consent of the Publisher, except brief quotes used in reviews.

Printed in the United States of America

Thanks to Dominique Wilkins of DW'S Graphics for the great cover.

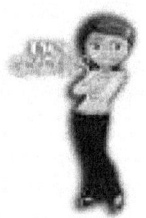

These stories are true. The names have been changed to protect the privacy of the individual and their families.

Table of Content

Introduction 7

Glossary 13

Cousin Flo 15

My Dear Brother 37

The Accident 57

Hip Deflated 75

The Red Flag 87

The Godgift 107

My Beautiful Daughter 127

Mr. Stone 139

An Exceptional Woman 155

The Mystery 167

Life Stockings 191

Honorable Toe 203

The Unwanted Guest 211

In A Blink Of An Eye 231

Conclusion 249

Introduction

As long as I can remember I always wanted to be a nurse. I don't know why. I had no role model. I never went to a hospital or even a doctor, never even met a real nurse. We lived in a very rural section of Mississippi and I was basically a very healthy child. My grandmother, who lived nearby, had a remedy for all our ills when we were sick. She was johnnie-on-the-spot with the "drink your milk lecture," and the "eat your greens" command, as well as the annual dose of chill tonic. Every ache and pain was credited to "growing pains."

I don't know how I knew what a nurse did. I must have heard talk about some nurse, maybe one who had saved the life of a neighbor or relative. Maybe I'd read a book from school library that inspired me.

We were fortunate to have a very progressive high school in our area that is it was advanced for that time. We had a well-equipped typing, shorthand, and bookkeeping department and I excelled in all of those courses. I could type 80 words a minute and could take 120 words a minute in shorthand. My grand plan was to become a secretary until I saved enough money to accomplish my goal of becoming a nurse.

After graduation from high school at the innocent age of 17, I set off to find the job that would eventually allow me to reach my goal. It didn't take long for me to realize that a girl such as I, even with my stellar school record, with my typing and shorthand speed was not going to be taken seriously. I tried my best to project a more sophisticated manner than I was capable of, and I'm afraid it showed. I was a country girl, a sharecropper's daughter, but I knew how to work. But I did not know anything about the city. We didn't even have electricity, indoor plumbing or running water in rural Neshoba County until I was 16 years old. We never had a telephone or television set as long as I lived at home.

It didn't take long for me to realize that I wasn't going to get very far in the staid business world of the early 50s. I could, however wait tables. That job needed quick hands and tough feet. I knew I could manage that. It helped that I was a people pleaser, and knew how to hold my real feelings behind a ready smile.

I went in pursuit of such a job. Employers looked me up and down and decided, yes indeed, I could handle this. Success and I started to work. I put on a confident face, which I knew was a pretty one. It had won the Neshoba County Beauty contest. I had naturally blond hair and blue eyes, there was always enough food on the table but I was fortune not to have an ounce of extra weight on my bones, but what I had was proportioned quite well, my grandmother said.

After three weeks of futile searching I gave up ever finding a job in Jackson. I packed up my things and moved to Pine Bluff, AK to live with my aunt. Trusting my luck would change. Not only did I get one job, I got two. I worked from 7 to 3 in one diner and then from 4pm to midnight at a drive in. It was fun and amusing because people kept telling me there was a girl who looked just like me working at a café just down the street. I learned to smile in a sly way, and dip my chin, and play innocent. Soon the smile became part of me and the more I smiled the more the customers' tips grew. Neither of my bosses ever knew I was working a second shift at a competing establishment.

    The money was good and the tips were better. Any penny or dime left at the end of the week went into my fruit jar savings for making my dreams come true. The days, so full of work, passed quickly and soon the jar was running over. Now I could see possibility and I worked more diligently than ever. My hard work finally paid off and off to nursing school I went.

After demanding work hours and long hours of studying I was able to obtain my nursing degree. There was not a break from the tough work but it has been worth it and very rewarding. God allowed me to be in the right place at the right time during my fifty difficult but rewarding years in Health Care. They were profitable and life changing. I thank God for the guidance and direction He has given me during these years.

Glossary

MED-MAL .... Medical Malfeasance

Baby Bringer .... Obstetrician Doctor
Baby Tender .... Pediatricians Doctor
Bone Fixers .... Orthopedic Surgeon
Bone Shop .... Orthopedic Clinic
Cat Bird Seat .... All under my control
Cutting Stitcher .... Surgeon
Cutting Stitching Table .... Operating Table
Godbody .... Doctor
Godgift .... Baby
Godhouse .... Hospital
Poison Passer .... Anesthesiologist
Stitching Helper .... Operating Room Technician

Life snuffed out far too soon, depriving two little girls of any memory of their mother.

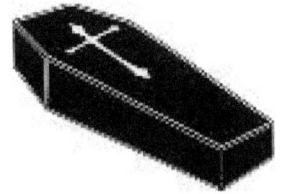

I don't always understand God's plan especially when it comprises of leaving two small girls without a mother.

Cousin Flo

Chapter 1

My cousin Flo was a very special person in my life. We were about the same age, both of us were blue eyed blondes, soulmates. We shared everything since we were thirteen and lived in Neshoba County in Mississippi. Now we were both pregnant. I was in my last three months and not doing well. My blood pressure and blood sugar were both running high with ten pounds of fluctuating edema. I was still working in the Cutting Stitching Shop, barely dragging my bloated, disfigured body home after ten to twelve hour shifts. I continued to drag because my dear Flo needed looking after.

Flo was in her ten to twelve week stage. They weren't sure which one because she had been bleeding since the beginning. She and her husband, Jack, had two precious little girls ages two and four.

Jack so desperately wanted a boy. It did not matter that they were hard pressed to feed, clothe and care for the two children they already had. Flo was a beautiful human being. She took her mother and wife roles very seriously, which is why she was pregnant again trying to have a son. Her Baby-Bringer had advised bed rest. This was to combat the bleeding and a special diet to try and control the awful nausea and vomiting that plagued her. Flo wasn't doing either very well. She couldn't stay off her feet. Jack would go to work all day leaving her to care for their two active little girls all alone. Jack said they couldn't afford to hire someone and Flo was not yet willing to ask family for help.

    When I saw her I could not believe my eyes. She was very pale, as "pale as a piece of cotton." I could see that she was also very weak by the way her hand trembled as she reached for the crackers that I had brought. This was her worse day yet. I was barely able to keep back the tears when I looked at my dear cousin friend. Though the windows were wide open, there was not a breath of fresh air in the room.

"What happened to the bed," I asked as I stared at the rumpled mess.

"Oh, the slat broke this morning. I didn't think I should try and lift the mattress, all things considered," she said while faintly smiling. "I figured it was better for my head to be down, anyway," she quipped.

"What have you had to eat today," I asked as I marveled about her upbeat spirit. I was sure I would not be in that kind of spirit in her situation. Then with a sad expression on her face, Flo said, "Jack left some juice and crackers by the bed when he left, but the girls ate them. That's ok because I wouldn't have been able to keep them down anyway."

"We have got to find a better way to handle this! You simply cannot go without eating. It's too dangerous," I said in a stern exasperated voice. I'm quite sure she picked up on that.

"I expect to do better," she said. Her blue eyes were smiling at me but her voice was very weak. "I've only bled a little today," she quickly added as if to take my mind off the food situation.

"Jack has got to get some help around here for a little while, or else I'm going to call your mother," I said again very sternly.

"He says he can't afford it. You know my mother has all she can juggle just taking care of her own problems." Flo was trying to reason with me. "Besides, he took me to the ER and I got two bottles of I.V. fluid yesterday and I feel a lot better." She then raised herself on her elbows and added. "I can't help it if the damned bed broke. I know how it looks to you, but I really am doing better." It was then that I seemed to see a little fire in her eyes.

"Alright then," I said while trying to not offend her anymore. Then I turned and sighed and grimaced at the same time. "But you better eat everything I brought you and keep it down. Now let me see if I can fix that cotton-picking slat for you," I said as I waddled to the foot of the bed to see what I could do. I was able to fix the slat before I had to go that day, but I still didn't feel happy about the situation she was in.

Chapter 2

I continued to check on Flo as often as I could. The bleeding finally stopped but she still had to go two or three times a week for I.V. fluid. The nausea and vomiting persisted. It was August and with the weather being so very hot dehydration proved to be a real threat.

Flo had chosen a Baby-Bringer that was known as a Cat-about-Town, a favorite with all the ladies. It didn't matter that his Cutting-Stitching ability was far less than the best, his bedside manner was rated a ten plus. "Let little mama have whatever little mama wants," he would always say. This seemed to be one of his favorite sayings. The little mamas eat it up too, taking full advantage of the situation. Never mind that what they wanted was not always what they needed.

He was a handsome devil, and was very involved in a steamy extra marital affair with a lady in white. This just seemed to increase his popularity.

His practice was booming and babies were everywhere. Until one day his less colorful partner pulled the rug out from under him. What a surprise that was. It seemed that there was a prepractice agreement signed by both that should either of them cause trouble or embarrass to the other in any way that the partnership would be automatically dissolved. Dissolved is just what happened the day the wife of the Cat-about-Town stormed into the office, full of little mamas, and screamed, "I am going to kill that slut in white who's sleeping with the father of my children!"

Pandemonium prevailed. The office split, records were getting transferred, there was confusion among the mamas, and gossip abounded. What a mess that clinic was in. I wondered how much of this disaster Flo knew. Also I wondered if Flo was getting lost in the shuffle and chaos of the clinic. I know that half the cure for a person having trouble is having faith in the healer, so I never relayed my concern to Flo. I was still a little miffed that she had not asked my opinion about this guy in the first place. I am a nurse and I know many of these doctors. I was glad that she was doing much better, but it would serve her right to get caught up in this entire hullabaloo, I thought more out of anger than lack of concern.

Chapter 3

I knew I needed to focus on myself. I felt that I was getting uglier and bigger by the day. My word, I thought, carrying this third Godgift is getting to be real burden. My health status did not improve. The antibody titer, which is the RH blood reaction to the positive blood, ran higher with each test which meant for sure that this child would have a real fight for survival at birth. Damn that RH factor! Preparation was made to induce my labor six weeks before the due date to stem the allergic reaction between mother and child. A complete blood exchange would be done immediately after birth. There would be no waiting for the results of a test that may or may not be reported correctly. All these things weighed heavy on my mind. I was able to maintain my sanity only by working so hard that it was impossible to think. I did this right up to the induction date.

It was the last day in September, a Monday morning, and the day of my induction had finally arrived. I was sitting at the dining room table going over last minute details with Mama regarding little Mary.

"Now Mama, Mary has been weaned, don't give her the bottle," I told her, and then said, exhibiting more assurance than I felt, "Everything is going to be just fine. Sunday's child is full of grace, Monday's child is fair of face' and we're going to have us a Monday child." I recited the old legend to help pull up our spirits and pretend I had no worries. "Maybe it will be a girl," I added

"I hope not," Mama replied, refusing to be cheered up. "Girls are nothing but headaches and heartaches."

"Well, from here on out everything is in somebody else's hands. All we can do is pray," I said out loud as I fumed inside.

Everything had gone just too well. Induction had gone smooth, labor had been easy, a beautiful boy-child had been born and the exchange transfusion had gone without a hitch. Friday came and I did not believe my luck. I was wishing now that some of my good luck could rub off on Flo. When I got home with little Mike and Mama told me that Flo had been admitted to the Protestant Godhouse with the flu. "Just in case of trouble," she said. Then added, "You know with her being pregnant and all."

"I'm glad she's where someone will see about her. Jack will live to regret leaving her with those children to fend for themselves with Flo in the shape she has been in," I said as I breathed a sigh of relief.

Chapter 4

Saturday morning little Mike began to have diarrhea and vomiting. I could not get him any relief throughout the whole day. By evening I had emptied my bag of tricks and the child was no better. His stool was now green and foul smelling. "Oh God," I cried as my senses reasoned and the shock of reality hit me square in the face, "it's baby-room staph infection."

Luck was not on my side when I found out my Baby-Tender was out of town. I had no faith in his on call partner. I had to phone him anyway. He informed me that he was down with the flu.

"I don't know what the baby's problem is but do you want me to see him and give him the flu on top of it?" He asked as he sniffed.

I reckoned not. I held little Mike close and whispered in his tiny ear "well, we're in for it, just you and me, kid."

Monday morning at six a.m. I was found holding Mike, pacing as I waited for the Baby-Tenders' office to open. Mike was as white as snow, his dark hair framing his beautiful little face made it look even whiter. He was flaccid, unresponsive and too weak to even cry. Thank God, Mike's Baby-Tender was the first to arrive at his office. We all went immediately to the Protestant Godhouse.

Mike weighed in at four and half pounds, four pounds less than his birth weight. Immediately I.V.'s were started, antibiotics for the Godhouse acquired staph infection, and sponge baths to lower the fever. I sat by his side around the clock and counted the I.V. drops until my eyes crossed. I sponged, caressed, even talked to my baby and slept when he did. I was his nurse as well as his mother. Nobody could sense things my baby needed and carry them out like I could, I was his mother and there I was going to stay. I felt that little Mike knew I was by his side. Nobody else could possibly have cared for him like me his caring and loving mother. I stood over his bed and watched him intensely, and when I sagged into a chair at his side, I prayed until sleep snatched me away. I quickly returned when I heard him stir.

My meals were sent up to the room from the cafeteria. No one but the Baby-Tender was allowed in the room. The door was not even opened for my husband Vic. Our baby and I were in isolation. I called Vic twice a day with an update. I was always trying to push aside my fears.

I would not even go one floor down to see Flo who had been admitted to the Godhouse when a regular blood test had shown her to be dangerously anemic. Her blood count was at six, when it should have been between twelve and fourteen. She had obviously bled more than she admitted. I felt my brain would explode during those sleepless nights. Every fiber of my being wanted to help my dear friend but I could not risk my child's life to do it. So there I sat by my son praying for his life.

Chapter 5

I counted the days as I sat there in the hospital. Five days had passed and little Mike had slowly started down the road to recovery. He started gaining weight and acquired a faint baby pink color. While Mike made progress, Flo sank into oblivion. By the time I felt I could leave Mike to check on her, it was too late.

I found her alone, unconscious in an oxygen tent, drowning in her own body fluid. Her flu had morphed into pneumonia. Her blood count was so low that her body never developed a fever to fight the infection. She died trying to have a son for her husband, a man who couldn't take care of the children he already had.

She also died because the Cat-about-Town never took the time to do a simple test that is done routinely on all pregnant women. It was a simple blood count. How hard would that have been? It is unthinkable that such a medical atrocity could be committed in this day and age.

    Flo died because she trusted her life to two men who couldn't manage their own. Flo's untimely, unnecessary death rested squarely on the shoulders of the two men she trusted the most. To this day my blood boils when I think of these two bastards. I fervently hope daily that they have suffered some way for what happened to my dear friend. I know Flo would want me to forgive those two, and maybe someday I will, but not today. I need more time. After all, it has only been thirty years and my heart still aches.

    Dear, precious forgiving, sweet Flo, I miss you every day more than words can even tell.

*He lived his life to the full.
I was his shadow!*

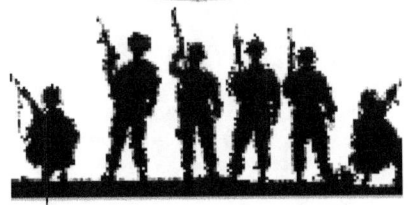

Some people have it their way not God's way.

MY DEAR BROTHER

Chapter 1

At birth my brother was named Garth Clifton by my mother. My father dubbed him Bill. He was called that all his life. He was the oldest of three children; therefore his lot was harder than the rest of us. He quit school in the tenth grade and got a job in the woods with a logging company. It was the only job available for the winter months. He did this to help support the family. In the summer he worked in the fields with the rest of us. I was his shadow and he took me with him everywhere he went. I was a tom-boy and he loved showing me off. I could shoot a rifle, ride a horse, swim fast and was somewhat a daredevil. I had the tallest pair of tom-walkers or stilts in the crowd, won every race.

He was tall, bright and handsome. He had those Pope blue eyes that crinkled when he smiled, what a smile. Lord the number of girls who were captivated by that smile. It seemed to say, "Come along with me," and they did! They didn't even seem to notice the slightly over-lapping eye tooth on the right. His physique was also a drawing point for the ladies. He had not one ounce of fat. He never dieted and when he started putting on weight he got busy and worked it off. He wanted to keep his great physique and his job, which was a hard one, helped him to stay in great shape.

    He continued his back-breaking work schedule, wood in the winter, fields in the summer until he was seventeen. At that point, he joined the army and became our savior. He sent money home to our poor, share-croppers house. My mother bought our first washing machine with some of the money. Oh what a blessing that was. The laundry was the hardest job to do, especially in the winter months. Other purchases we were able to make due to my brothers willingness to support us was a refrigerator, electric lights and eventually a bicycle for my younger brother and me.

Chapter 2

He lived his life loose, blaming it on his lack of education. During his service he had six wives, or live-ins, during his time in the service. He only had one child in spite of his many relationships. One day, while stationed in Japan he had a terrible wreck on a motorcycle. He was unconscious for a week. He had multiple fractures to his right leg and stayed in the hospital eighteen months. After that time he came home on leave to continue his recovery. He arrived home with his right leg in a cast that came up to his waist. The fact that he could not drive did not slow him down. I gladly drove him all over the country side with his leg hanging out of the door of that old GMC pick-up truck.

After he recovered, he went back to Japan at which time he had a Japanese girlfriend. He felt sorry for her and her family because they didn't have much. One day he gave them a bar of soap from the Commissary. Even though it was not war time, this was forbidden. My brother ended up getting caught and was given a dishonorable discharge. After that, he came home.

Chapter 3

When he came home he got a job building small motors at the local motor plant. He worked there for twenty years. While working there he had several gall bladder attacks; however he kept going. After battling this for a time, he had to have it removed. All seemed to be going well. On the second day Dick and I had decided to go visit my other brother, Mike, in Virginia.

We were having a great time visiting Mike when we arrived. The next day we got a call from May, Bills' currant wife. She was terribly shaken and told us we needed to come because Bill was still in the hospital and had taken a turn for the worse. We threw our things in the suitcase and off we went. We drove all night because this was no small trip.

Chapter 4

When we arrived at the hospital we found Bill in bed blown up like a balloon. After talking to him we found out they had done everything imaginable to him, including enemas, x-rays, tubes and other tests. Nothing they did helped the situation that Bill was in. I automatically thought it was pain from a buildup of gas from complications from earlier surgery and he just needed to get up and walk. He did just that. He walked and walked, despite the horrific pain. He did it like a solider, without complaint.

They had talked about them going back in. I knew that this would kill him considering the limited resources at this hospital. They were not equipped to deal with this kind of complicated severity. I did not hesitate to call a surgeon I knew. He had trained at the University when I was there and was practicing in a town close by. I picked up the phone called him and explained the situation. After talking for just a few brief moments, he directed us to bring Bill ASAP. We called an ambulance to pick him up and transport him to the hospital in Jackson, MS. We broke all the speed limits on our trip. We arrived at the emergency room, where my friend was practicing and hurried Bill right inside. My friend was there waiting. He laid his hand on Bills horribly swollen belly and said "take him directly to the operating room." He briefly greeted me assuring me they would take care of my brother and was off.

    Dick, May and I sat in the waiting area, where I paced the entire time. The surgeon finally came from the surgery room to talk to us. He talked to us very frankly about what had happened during the previous operation. He said the surgeon had left a "Silver Clip" across the common bile duct. This had stopped the flow of the bile that the liver always secreted. When the gall bladder is removed, the common duce is attached to the small bowel. The bile had backed up above the silver clip so much that the duct had perforated, spilling raw bile into Bills' abdomen. I was shocked!

Then I was distraught with myself that I had made him walk down the hall. All I knew was that he was swollen and in awful pain. My intent was good but result not so good. The terrible unthinkable pain he must have been in as we walked with bile pouring into his abdominal cavity. I had to shake myself to listen to the next words coming from the doctors' mouth. He said "I cannot promise you anything. It will all depend on his reaction to what had been done." We knew the next few days would be crucial and that they were. We could finally breathe easier when the life threating event was over. My surgeon friend told us that he would be glad to testify if we decided to pursue this atrocity. We did sue. We won and Bill was able to gain some monetary payment for the horrible nightmare he went through due to that physician's gross incompetence.

Chapter 5

When he had recuperated we resumed planting a garden across the road from his trailer. It was a beautiful garden. People in the community stopped along the road to admire it. It was a real show place and colorful, tomatoes, peppers of all colors red, green, yellow and purple. We also had yellow and white squash, zucchini and egg plants green and purple. That was not all Bill decided to grow a special watermelon. He picked the kind he wanted then he petted, watered and fertilized it just at the right times. At the end of its growth it weighed one hundred and ten pounds. We packed it up and took it to the Nursing Home where our mother lived. She was surprised at the great size. Then we had the best watermelon party ever, it was even written up in the local paper.

When he was able to return to work he went back to the motor plant. I called him on my way to work at Grenada the next night to see how things were moving along. To find out he had been in the local doctor's office most of the day. He was extremely dizzy to the point he couldn't even drive himself home from work. The doctor said it was vertigo and had him on a medication. The next morning he came into the kitchen for coffee. He fell hard in the middle of the floor. I again stepped in and had him come to Jackson to see a doctor here. I met him at my doctors' office I wanted to hear what was going on. He laid a stethoscope on Bills left carotid artery, no sound, the artery was completely occluded. Right then he was admitted to the hospital. He had surgery, a left carotid indarectomy was done. Problem solved and another sigh of relief.

Chapter 6

By this time Bill had retired. May had also left him, taking half of what he had plus all of his saving bonds. She came into the marriage with only the clothes on her back and left a wealthy woman. How sad. He was all alone. I spent as much time as I could with him, which was not a lot some weeks.

Our garden continued to be the talk of the community. His work ethic also never swayed. He kept himself busy not only with the garden but he did lawn care at several offices. As usual on a Sunday morning he was working at an office building mowing grass, planting flowers and just making the place look beautiful when he was attacked with stomach pain. He fell over and was taken to the local hospital. I called his son to inform him what was going on. He went to the hospital and sat with his dad. He was there three days with no diagnosis but the projectile of vomiting continued. I insisted his son bring him to Jackson.

They arrived by ambulance to the emergency room. There he stayed in and out of consciousness and in severe pain for six hours. We were waiting for the surgeon on call to arrive. Those few hours seemed like days. When he finally came at six o'clock that night the decision was to keep Bill overnight. He would stay in the intensive care unit overnight and have surgery the next morning. That is what happened. They found he had an intestinal stroke and his belly was full of dead colon. He had waited too long to come to the Jackson hospital causing too much of the colon to die to be removed. The decision by the surgeon to wait overnight before doing surgery had compounded the situation also. I knew at the sound of all this information that the outcome was not going to be a good one.

Chapter 7

As I sat with my brother my heart was gripped with grief as I watched him slipping away. He was unconscious. One time he regained consciousness long enough to ask me one last question. "Is this worse than the last time?" I hated to tell him the truth but I felt I must. I said "Yes, it is, Bill. You need to pray." Then he drifted off again. I trust he took that time to make things right with God but only God knows. I never got to talk to him again. The one thing I do know is that I dearly miss my brother. The garden that we created together just didn't mean as much after he died. The joy of it died. The garden also died because of lack of care. It has been many years since his passing, my heart still aches for his presences. I can still smell the coffee he would make at our house when he would come in the early morning hours. The aroma would wake me. I would rise from my bed with a smile on my face knowing he was there waiting to talk. Rest is peace my dear brother Bill, I love you.

Problems are forever present

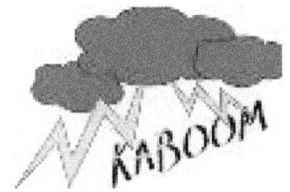

This would have taken me God, but I guess you weren't ready for me just yet. I understand that now.

THE ACCIDENT

Chapter 1

I was in my "hey day". I was young, had that country cornflower flavor, blonde hair, blue eyes and "stacked". I had even participated in several beauty contests, winning one in my senior year. After school I worked, scrimped, scratched and clawed my way through nursing school. It took me five years. Just two years out, I was in charge of the operating room at the local hospital. I called it the Godhouse because we hold people's lives in our hands. I was running the operating room in the very best Godhouse in the state, possibly in the South. The candidates who came for services were not always in agreement but what did they know? We all know when you were the receiving end of this business it was never pleasant. I knew that my Cutters and Stitchers (doctors) were the best because they were proficient in all the required disciplines. I only worked with the best.

Those ten to twelve hour days were a breeze for me. I had grown up the daughter of a share cropper, hard work and I became friends a long time ago. The work was always there from dawn to dusk, now was no different. But this job brought satisfaction. I was in control! The pay was excellent and I literally arranged the lives of all the helpers, consumers and the deliverers of my services. Those electric sliding doors and the pads always soaked with antiseptic protected my world and all who entered came at my invitation.

Every soul who presented themselves for service in my shop would get the very best. It did not matter that they could not appreciate the effort that went into the repair of their broken bodies. I knew they got the best and that is what counted. I never believed in doing only enough to get by. I always gave one hundred percent, it was like a cloud hovering over my head reminding me that my best was the only thing I could do.

"There is no minor surgery if it is being done on you," I often told the Stitching Helpers when they complained about being assigned to the minor stitching room. I guarded my precious supplies like a drill sergeant. You would think the money came out of my pocket, was said to me many times. To this I replied "it does yours too, if you pay taxes or have stitching insurance."

Chapter 2

I thought of each day like Christmas! I never knew what was inside the package until it was opened. That is exactly how it is with the patients that come through our doors. The excitement of this stress overload, fast paced, life and death game had to be experienced to be fully appreciated! The chief of the Poison Passers was the only player that shared the control of my world. I called the anesthesiologist, Poison Passer because if too much is given it becomes poison and it can kill. But it was necessary, after all, broken pieces could not be repaired or new parts put in without the pain-blocking poison that his flock peddled. What a joy it was to work with him. He was tall, dark, and handsome in its original concept, none better. We considered each other brilliant. What a formidable team we posed for the Cutting and Stitching Godbodies. If there was no Poison Passer available, no case, if there was no room, no stitching helpers, ditto. He was like the Jitterbug (dance) King and I loved to dance.

Every day I was in the Cat Bird seat, the one in control, but come Christmas the seat got lined with red velvet. My chief Cutter-Stitcher gave me the honor of planning the party for the shop! He provided a room at the Country Club; the rest was up to me. To this point it had been the bash of the year, especially the time one of our boy Poison Passers put one hundred percent alcohol in the punch fountain. Even the Chief cut a rug that night.

This year I decided I would put my stitching helpers in the lime light. We would dream up some radical costume and do a chorus line. Strictly volunteer participation. I was the first to sign up. I now had to find fifteen pairs of shoes that were exactly alike raging in sizes from five to eleven that were danceable. After a diligent search I was able to find them in two different stores down-town. I arranged to meet another chorus girl, Abbie, at one of the stores to get a much needed second opinion.

Chapter 3

I arrived at the store early as was my nature. I decided to walk across the street to the store to make sure they had held the shoes as I had requested. I carefully surveyed the traffic. A line of cars were stopped in the right turn lane. A considerate male driver motioned me to pass. I smiled my thanks, looked to the left and saw two vacant lanes, I was now in the center of the six lane street. Looking to my right for oncoming traffic, a noise caused me to look again down the two previously empty lanes. Oh no, a car had pulled out of the turn lane, crossed over the second lane and was headed straight for me. FAST!!! After some split second thinking, I decided I'll jump on the hood because I don't want to be caught under the wheels. On impact I flew through the air at least twenty feet up and thirty feet down the street. My purse went one way and me the other. People were screaming. I landed flat on my butt and skidded six feet on the asphalt. I was so embarrassed, my dress above my waist, stockings torn, and my shoes gone. I attempted to get up but I couldn't move my left leg, major damage. There I had to sit, and then the alligator tears began to come. I couldn't even think about what to do. Every store in the area must have called an ambulance. I could hear them coming and see the lights flashing. "I must decide which Godhouse before they picked me up" I thought. I wanted desperately to go to my own, with the help of my Chief and my devoted cutting and stitching trainee. There I could direct my own care, control my destiny. The traffic was tied up for hours.

    My mind raced with the assessment of damages telling me that repair would have to be done in the bone shop. That was the kicker. I just couldn't face being spread-eagled on that instrument from hell called the fracture table. Forget about the modicum of dignity afforded in the other shop where only the part to be repaired was exposed. In this shop it all hung out. No help for it.

The picture I had in my head was not a pretty one both feet tied to metal slabs, arms attached to boards, back and butt on small wooden supports. I would be totally suspended in mid-air, not a stitch of cover, a wooden pole jammed between my legs to keep me that way. Why did they have to take x-rays during the repair anyway? I questioned as I saw the whole undignified scene play out in my head. I knew the x-ray was necessary but that did not change the fact that I was not happy about it. No, I decided I would not be "hung on that cross" where I would know everybody in the room. I could hear the ambulance pulling up, it was okay because I had a plan.

Chapter 4

"Which hospital do you prefer?" the ambulance driver enquired.

"Take me to the Training Godhouse," I told the driver "and wait for the x-rays. If surgery has to be done I want to go to the Protestant Godhouse." They understood completely and did as I instructed. I laid there waiting for my arrival at the hospital to find out the whole awfulness of my situation. A short ride seemed like forever.

The chief of the Bone Shop arrived, after assessing the situation he informed me that the x-rays showed no open repair of the hip was needed. Then he told me of his plan of treatment put me to bed, and apply traction to both feet. I was notified that it was twenty pounds for each foot. I was sure they made a mistake and put forty pounds from the way it felt. The mattress had a board under it and the usual plastic cover. The hip didn't hurt, but oh my, what a number that plastic cover did on my brush-burn butt! What a predicament I was in.

    I pressed the button for the nurses to help with the bed pan and waited until I thought I was going to explode. Then I took matters in my own hands. It was definitely a major problem. I almost ended up hanging by my feet several times just trying to get it out of the bedside stand. Then the nurses finally came to assist me, and then left the room. Then it was the problem of them coming to take it away. When no one came to empty it I was greatly tempted to dump it on the floor. The bed pan was definitely my number one enemy. It was necessary, but inconvenient and that's not to mention the indescribable pain when the cold steel met my brush-burn.

    Meal times were the only bright spot in the monotonous days. The Food Person that delivered my food was only to deliver it not serve it. That meant wherever the tray in my room was that is where they set my food. They did not move the tray close to my bed, they left it just out of my reach. What was I supposed to do? Get out of bed and get it? That was impossible. I had to wait until someone brought it within reach. By the time I got to it a bad meal had turned god-awful. I think the Food Person should have to lay down in the bed unable to move and see what an impossible task it is to reach the food when they put so far away. They might think twice where they placed trays after that.

Chapter 5

I deduced two major conclusions from this experience. First, all Godbodies and Helpers needed to spend at least forty-eight hours in traction, ideally with a brush-burn on their back side. Then they would understand better how their patients felt, and they might even have a little more sympathy. The second conclusion was the food service shop was very disorganized and not patient friendly. They couldn't hold a candle to the way my Cutting and Stitching rooms were run, which was very smoothly.

I got out of the Godhouse on the day of the Christmas party. I was still hobbling around on crutches, couldn't even wear one shoe. But I got decked out in a new outfit anyway. I was determined to go and enjoy myself as best I could in my condition. Off I went with a smile on my face.

I was met at the car by my wonderful resident. He carried me in his arms into the party room. Everyone cheered and toasted me as I entered the room. This was the highlight! Then the show began. House lights dimmed, music started, and the Cutting and Stitching Rocketters skipped out on stage. The spot lights shinned right through the costume material, thirty breasts bounced, along with nipples of various shapes and sizes jiggling and showing clearly, and fifteen pubic hair patches were on prominent display. Abbie really was a natural blond after all. The audience gasped, but the Rocketters danced, oblivious to the display they were giving. The house came down, the Rocketters thought they were a great success. It is a show no one will forget that is for sure. This was to be the only time in my life I was truly thankful not to be in the spot-light. To this day I don't think they know what it really meant for them to be in the spot light that night.

Be careful of greener pastures, they might not be so green.

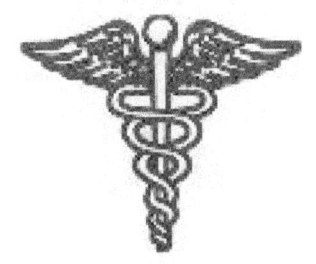

God touched the hands of the surgeons to perform a perfect surgery and then he blessed the rehab.

Hip Deflated

Chapter 1

Years passed and the once fractured hip gradually started to crumble. I knew I had to make a decision but the positioning on that torture device, the fracture table still haunted me. There is just no other way to do it. So I finally made the decision to just go ahead and do it. Meanwhile, I happened to catch a program on television from Vanderbilt in Nashville TN. Lo and behold they had perfected a procedure for hip replacement that involved a small incision of three inches as opposed to the six inches one routinely did at the local Godhouse. This would shorten my stay on the torture table and lesson my rehabilitation time.

I eagerly made contact with Vanderbilt and learned that the bone fixers name was Dr. Shanen. I quickly made an appointment and off to Nashville I went to sign up for this new hip procedure. I was very anxious to get this done. I could hardly walk. It would take me away from family. I wouldn't know a soul involved. Oh boy lots of stress gone!

I got everything scheduled. Cutting day came, husband, cousins, Joe and Phillip, were all present. All went well. I guess I was in my room with the catheter in place and I immediately demanded it be removed, which they did. When I stood up catheter residue, blood and mucous, plopped out on the floor, my husband wiped it up with a paper towel the best he could and called for a nurse. This cleaning procedure required special cleaning with Clorox. Nobody came except a covey of bone fixers led by my chief. I tried to tell them that they were standing on contaminated ground but no one was listening. They left carrying by blood and mucous all over the Godhouse.

Chapter 2

Cutting and stitching and my new hip occurred on Friday. Plans were made to move me to the getting well building on Saturday. This was a beautiful structure, oh boy I was moving up in the world. There were a number of other victims in various stages of survival. They all were on blood thinners as was usual for these types of cutting. One was recovering from a lung transplant.

Chapter 3

"Hello, my name is Mitsi Brown. I am your physical therapist." The lady said as she entered my room on Sunday afternoon. Also that she would be seeing me in that department. She left the room but failed to tell me where the department was and how I was to get there. After she left I slowly got up and attempted to find my way to that department. It was way down the hall. When I entered, Mitsi, the physical therapist, proceeded to give me a thorough work out, lateral, normal leg lift's, etc. I dragged my new painful hip, tired leg and aching back to my room, in search of relief. I was in extreme need of rest.

Monday morning came and everything was a buzz. The head nurse came into my room, introducing herself and deposited a wheel chair in my room. "What is that for," I quizzically asked. Her reply was "to take you to physical therapy." "Well I walked down there yesterday," I said. "Oh my, well someone will come and get you in a while," was her reply. "I want to ask you a favor," I pleaded. "Would you take a look at my incision site? It feels funny." I lifted my robe to give her access to the area. She paled I thought she was going to faint. She said, "Get in bed now! The doctor has to see this." What she saw was a hematoma about the size of a grapefruit at the incision site. It was an unwanted present from the physical therapy treatment. The attending bone tender came, "well this is very unfortunate, but there is nothing we can do, but to keep quiet. No walking or therapy for a few days." He wanted me to keep quiet so no one would know their blunder. He didn't say but I heard that this blunder would delay my healing. It did!!!

Chapter 4

After three days, I started walking and the death stocking battle began. The established procedure for these items were stocking on during the day, off during the night. This was exactly reversed to what I had been taught. Common sense would tell you that pressure was needed when you were still, not during activity. The difficulty of these awful things was that you could not get them back on once they were taken off and off they came at night by caregiver.

About the forth morning, as was expected, my left leg was swollen and red. I couldn't put the stockings back on. The resident bone tender confirmed the catastrophe. Yes a blood clot. Off I went to the Godhouse for confirmation, a Doppler was done and, thank God it was a superficial blood clot, not deep which was the traveling type.

I was so angry!! Not a word was said on the way back to restoration "nightmare". We arrived just as lunch was being served. All were gathered and on every plate was a large clump of broccoli. We had several green things served but never this. I picked mine up and threw it across the room and yelled "I want to see the dietitian." She came, a young visibly upset lady. "Where did you go to school?" I demanded. "Everybody walking down the street knows you don't give greens to people who are on anticoagulants or commonly known as blood thinners. This lady over here has had a lung transplant. Green things are high in Vitamin K. What do think a clot would do to her?" I berated. She just stood there with fear in her eyes saying, "I am sorry, so sorry." She left. I choose my meals from then on. I don't know what happened to the rest of those poor souls on that mistake, hidden restoration nightmare.

Chapter 5

The next day I called my daughter and told her to come and get me before they killed me. She and my daughter-in-law arrived that day to take me home. We left and with the wheel chair in tow, we were taken to the airport. We were loaded on the plane with full knowledge that it was not recommended that I fly so soon after the cutting. I made the decision to risk the flight. I would rather risk flying than to threaten my life with another episode at the Restoration Center. I came home and set up my own Restoration Center. Thank God all came out blessed.

*A life well lived,
she fought the
good fight.
She doubled my
joy, divided my
grief.
I miss her!!!*

She left this world in agony but was relieved when she was received into God's hand.

THE RED FLAG

Chapter 1

My childhood friend, Jo, and I were going to Rome, the Eternal City. Two girls from Neshoba County, MS were going to take it all in. The last time I was in Rome, I vowed to take Jo with me the next time I went. Jo had never been outside of Neshoba County until she met and married Phillip and moved to Decatur, Alabama. She always wanted to see Rome's churches.

Jo and I had grown up helter-skelter with my Grammie as our grounding rock. Jo's mother was Grammie's sister. She died when Jo was six months old. Jo stayed with Grammie; and her two older sisters went to Belzoni with her father's family. Jo did not see her sisters until she was twelve years old, then again when they were adults. They could not visit because there was a transportation problem.

You see they did not have a car and all their traveling was by horse and wagon. Grammie and I were her family.

We were closer than most sisters, with her silver blond hair and snappy green eyes. We even looked like sisters. She was full of mischief and always up to something. She'd say, "Aw, let's just do it! Grammie won't care." We would steal eggs and bury them in the sawdust pile to let the sun cook them while we looked for grapes, muscadine, or huckleberries to eat with them. It took about two hours to cook the eggs, depending on how deep we had buried them.

One day when Jo and I were engaged in some such activity, her father, Claude, spotted us. He was in the field plowing with the oxen. He must have thought we were just playing. He stilled his team, broke a switch from a plum tree on the fence line and came after us. Just that morning we had gone through a thicket of shumac bushes. As it turned out Jo was allergic to them and broke out in hot blisters all the way up to her drawers. When her dad, came at us with his switch, he laid into Jo. He lashed her legs with keen branch from the plum tree until blood ran down her already blistered legs. This was only an example of all the horrors that he perpetrated over the years. He lived with Grammie and Papa Pope. They felt helpless to intervene, after all, she was his child and he had control.

When he was done I grabbed Jo's arm and helped her all the way to Grammies'. She was appalled. Her face was stern and she was near tears as she ran to get a can of lard. She laid Jo on a quilt on the floor and cleaned the blood away. Grammie used the lard as a healing agent. It was like ointment and would keep the infection away. She applied the lard to soothe the injuries on her legs.

Chapter 2

Jo and I did a lot of chores around the farm, and once we were finished at our place we were hired out to members of the community. We chopped cotton, thinned corn, picked butterbeans and in the fall before school started, we picked cotton. These were just a few things we were required to do, both at home and for others. We did whatever was needed, and we did it all for a dollar a day or board. We knew the people so we stayed with them as long as they needed our help. When Jo was in the tenth grade she dropped out of school and moved to Laurel. She lived with her aunt. That is where she met Phillip and got married.

After we were grown, I was able to visit Rome and see all it beautiful, magnificent treasure. I knew this was a place Jo had to see and I vowed to take her with me one day. That day finally came and we were ready for all the glory of this ancient city.

Chapter 3

When we arrived we wasted no time hitting the streets. We dropped coins in the Trevi Fountain, stared at the beauty of Saint Peters, and walked the steps of the two thousand year old Coliseum. We knew those walls held many secrets. Our next attraction was St. Paul's Outside the Walls, with its great, green marble columns, and the two priceless glowing green malachite altars which sat one on either side of the mail altar.

The next day we were going to Tivoli, east of Rome, to tour Villa d'Este and its majestic water gardens and fountains. Cardinal d'Este built this in the tenth century by harnessing a natural river. This is an engineering feat that could not be duplicated today. Tourism promotes a spot in the d'Este gardens where there is a fountain on either side of the walkway which forms an arch of water over the walkway. According to legend, you are supposed to be able to walk under the arch and not get a drop of water on your head. I know that this is true because I have walked this way before. I couldn't wait to be with Jo when she saw it. While we were standing in the gardens of Villa d'Este, taking in all the beautiful surroundings, I couldn't help but be haunted by the words Jo had whispered to me. After taking in all its beauty, Jo and I decided to start getting ready for the trip, by car, to Sicily the next day.

"This trip is making me young again." Jo said as the sun came up while we were standing on the street waiting for the car. She was flushed with excitement.

"How so?" I asked.

"I've just started my period again!" She whispered as she pulled me away from the crowd.

"Jo." I said with dismay as a cold chill went up my spine. "You are seventy years old and this is not a good sign." I made her promise that as soon as we got home she would go and see her doctor. "This is not something you put off," I said with a great sternness.

In spite of this cloud hanging over us, we had a wonderful day. Jo wanted to see all of the beautiful churches. She was a devout Christian and had no vices; she was well read on the Bible and "believed every jot and tittle there in." She was the best person I have ever known.

Our magical time in Rome was coming to an end. We packed our bags, and a boatload of camera shots, and prepared for our flight home.

Chapter 4

When we were back home, unpacked and back in our routines, I called Jo and asked if she'd gone to the doctor. She answered that she had and that he did not do anything. "We'll watch things for now," he said.

"Go to another doctor," I strongly advised her.

"But this one goes to our church. I have confidence in him," she responded.

I felt my hands were tied. What could I do? Months had passed before another call. I took a deep breath and picked up the phone to call Jo again to see what was being done about her health. Her doctor had sent her to an OB-GYN doctor. "Thank God," I said to myself with a sigh of relief.

"My boobs are so sore," she said as we talked.

"Why!" I yelled at her.

"Oh," she paused like she was scared of me, "he put me on hormones."

"Get off of them!" I screamed. I couldn't believe this. "Get off right NOW! Get yourself to another doctor. This one is crazy!" Every fool walking the street knows that a vaginal bleed in someone over seventy years old is a strong warning sign of cancer. I knew hormones would feed cancer, if she had it. We ended the conversation with her promising she would go back to the doctor.

She did go back to the doctor. They decided now they would do a D&C procedure, which is scraping out the uterus of its contents. Jo did not get any better. Finally a decision was made to have a hysterectomy. As far as I was concerned this was a year late in being done. This should have been done at the onset.

Jo was not sharing the results of the pathology report with me so off to Decatur, Alabama I went. Fear of what I would find gripped me as I drove to Jo's house. My dear friend, I thought with tears in my eyes.

After I arrived and greeted my dear friend with the usual hug, we did some small talk. It wasn't long before I insisted in looking at the pathology report. When I saw it, my heart stopped for a second, as I read the words: **cervical cancer**. I could hardly keep the tears from flowing down my cheeks. Jo smiled at me and told me the doctor said, "This little old tumor is no bigger than that of a pencil lead." This was of no comfort to me because they did not mention that there were five positive nodes in the pelvis. The doctors had not explained anything, much less what it would mean for Jo. It had been two years since Rome, no pap-smear had been done, and this "little old tumor" had spread. A pap smear would have at least been one way of ruling out cervical cancer.

Chapter 5

Treatment was now to begin. She did not respond well to the chemo. It caused her to vomit until she could no longer walk. Then they tried radium. The vomiting continued unabated and her belly swelled. She had grown another tumor while on treatment, a tumor so big it caused an obstruction in her colon. Surgery had to be done to relieve the obstruction. I knew then she was doomed. Sadness filled my whole being.

The treatment was not over. They place a radium implant in her vagina. This procedure had been abandoned thirty years ago. Again her suffering was unimaginable. No one could go near her while this was being done. It was because the radium treatment put out a lot of rays and it was not good for people to be around. This treatment had been discontinued years before but they were doing it to Jo. She was all alone, except the God to whom she prayed continually.

Chapter 6

Still trusting in her doctor, she went to hospice at their instruction. Jo thought that was just another kind of treatment. The whole time she thought she was going to get better, she had not realized what hospice really was. At last her suffering was tempered, but not the vomiting. The next time I saw her, she was in a semi-private room. There was just a skeleton of a person left. She was bald and gaunt, but her everlasting spirit glowed in those precious green eyes.

I was not happy with the room situation. When I question it, I found out Medicare would not pay for a private room. I went to the business office and paid the difference. They moved her to a private room. I felt my dear friend deserved privacy while dying.

I knew she could not eat much. But I had a beautiful garden so I brought her a basket full of veggies because I knew she enjoyed tomatoes sandwiches. That was the last thing she ate before she died.

Jo was almost a perfect woman in my eyes. Her faith in God never wavered but mine was sorely tested during her illness. It puzzled me, and yes, angered me that God would allow her to suffer then take her. God has a reason for all things but at that moment I did not understand what it was, all I knew was my heart was broken I was missing my dear friend, Jo.

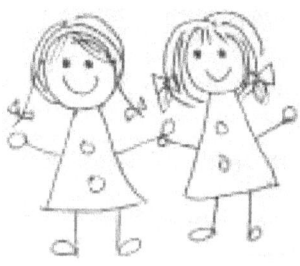

Born with a
fight to win,
so she did!!

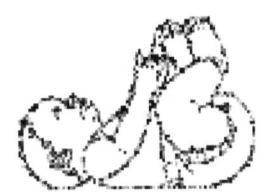

God blessed me with a beautiful baby girl. She had to fight a hard battle but won!!!

THE GODGIFT

Chapter 1

I was absolutely miserable. I was about as pregnant as anyone could be. My belly poked out, my belly button stuck out, and my ankles were twice their normal size. I was also tipping the scales at one hundred sixty five pounds, thirty pounds overweight. The Baby-Bringer had told me to exercise. It was beginning to be August where it would be ninety degrees in the shade. Where did he think I was going to exercise in this heat and what kind did he have in mind? I could barely walk! I was doing fine until about nine days ago, when at the Stitching Shop house, where I worked, everything seemed to have gone to hell in a hand cart. That is when I realized I had lost a lot of my mobility and my working days were numbered. I didn't have time to have this second baby anyway. My career was on the rise and everything was going my way, now this pregnancy. I hadn't planned on the first one and this one was just as much of a surprise. Little did I know that I would be blessed with child number two. I should have known not to trust Mr. Rhythm, Dick never could dance. I may as well make the best of it because there was no need to cry now. I was twenty weeks from delivery and was wondering if I would be blessed enough to have another child, as independent, brilliant and cute as my three year old son, Dick. He was early walking, talking and knowing what he wanted to do. My old heart just skipped a beat when he looked at me with those big brown beautiful eyes and said "youse a good boy mommy". He was returning a compliment I gave him when he was particularly on his good behavior. Now this one would be a brat, probably dumb too. This first one seemed to have gotten all the brains collectively that Dick and I had. Would be nice to have the girl Dick wanted. If she was pretty enough she wouldn't have to worry about being real smart. I would live to regret these thoughts from my tired suffering pregnant mind.

Chapter 2

Today was Saturday, August 9, 1953, and I in my tormented state, had to find a way to get through this day. My mother had come to be with me for this blessed event. She almost drove me crazy with her "don't do this, don't do that, you might mark the baby" words always coming from her mouth. I just wished she would shut up and that this baby would hurry and make its entrance into the world. I was tired of carrying it around with me. I thought that if I did house cleaning my mother would help, that would give us both something to do to pass the time. I started with the window blinds boy did they need it, next the hard wood floors, dry mop, wax and drag out the buffer. At least you could tell when this floor got done it shone like new money. Now since the blinds were clean I decided that the wood slates at the top could use a coat of paint. This really sent my mother into orbit.

"Don't smell the turpentine, it will send you into labor" my mother plucked.

Chapter 3

Good, I thought, anything to get this show on the road, something please. Bed time came and I did not want to think about tomorrow. I hauled my unrecognizable body into bed. Stretched out and all hell broke loose. Whoosh a lot of something warm and wet between my legs. God, no I am peeing on myself. Then the first labor pain hit hard. Hallelujah time to fly. Dick hadn't gone to bed yet and the suit case had been packed for a week. We were going so fast I thought we were air born. The seat of my house coat was wet and I didn't care now that I knew what it was. About half way to the hospital another pain, it felt like my whole belly was on fire, the muscles in my back started to go downward into my pelvis. Brother this Godgift is in a mighty big hurry to travel down the Birth Canal Street. I demanded Dick to step it or did he want to deliver the baby right here and now. We arrived at the Protestant Godhouse and went straight to the Baby

Getting Shop. We had called ahead to the ER to apprize them of our arrival. I was met by the evening super gale. This was Miss Hotty Totty today. She looked like she had been weaned on a pickle and didn't know shit from Shinola (shoe polish).

She strolled up to the stretcher while putting on a pair of gloves. "I am going to examine you" she said.

"Ah, no you don't!" I yelled just as another gut wrenching, intense, evacuating pain hit. Just look under the cover and you will see why.

"Oh God she is crowning" screeched Miss Hotty Totty. "What color is its hair?" I panted as they flew down the hall to the Baby Dropping Room. The Baby Getter arrived on the scene just in time to catch little beautiful Mary as she made her entrance into the world. Man three pains that's the way to have them I thought as I drifted off and knowing Miss Hotty Totty didn't get the pleasure of examining me or hacking off my pubic hair. "Hot dam," I chuckled, "I showed all of them how babies should be born no enema, no probing in her private parts and no prep, just three pains and pop them out."

Chapter 4

I woke to find my bottom feeling as though it had done battle with a chain saw. I was altogether deflated and that felt good. At seven a.m. the partner of my choice and the baby tender came around and told me, "You have a beautiful baby girl." I breathed a sigh of relief because everything is just fine. That meant that the test that had been done for the RH factor had been negative. I was RH negative and Dick was positive opposites in every way. We had been told with the first baby that this might be a problem, with the second one and for sure the third one. Therefore the Coomb test would be done just to be sure. I was also told that should the test be positive that a complete blood exchange would have to be done on the child. I knew that this was a risky procedure and felt that weight had been lifted off me.

The head of the specimen testing lab came on duty at seven a.m. She saw the blood that had been taken from my child, the serum was yellow. She checked to see if the baby had had an exchange transfusion. To her bone chilling discovery she found that there had been no exchange. The report I had been given was in error. She set about to notify my chosen Baby Tender. Something must be done and now! Meanwhile the Baby Tender had come over to examine his newborns as was his custom. He took one look at our child's eyes said this baby is jaundiced, run another Coombs test. The lab chief found him in the nursery and informed him of the mistake. He came flying into my room, checks flushed, and breathing hard. I took one look at the routinely laid back man and knew immediately that something was terribly wrong. "How much do you know?" He asked me. I replied, "I haven't seen her yet." "Then you don't know anything," he replied.

Chapter 5

With that he proceeded to tell me about the wrong report. Also he said that the exchange would have to be done immediately. He also said if the exchange wasn't done within the first twelve hours of life that there is a better than average possibility that the child would be mentally retarded. That is if she lived at all. Of course I knew all this because I had helped with many exchange transfusions that was done in my cutting and stitching shop. I also knew the risk involved. My world turned dark grey, my thoughts chaotic. I knew the blood sucker that ran the test, that cocky chauvinistic bastard. I saw him in my mind's eye scratching his balls and yawning while he ran the test that meant life or death for my child. To him it was no big deal just another test to be run at four a.m.

The procedure was done, the waiting began. We decided to officially name our daughter Mary according to age old Italian custom. All first sons and daughters are named from the father's parents. Little Mary began the fight for survival. She was not only allergic to her father's RH factor, which caused her problem in the first place, but she developed another allergy to the type of blood used for the transfusion. She systematically started breaking down all the new red blood cells that had been given her. The fight and waiting continued well into the third day. I had not yet seen Mary but I was totally engulfed in the fight. I somehow felt that if I concentrated my whole being, body, mind and soul, hard enough that Mary would feel it. My force of energy would help her fight harder. This went on for four days. Mary became more jaundice turning a darker shade of yellow. Her "ectris index" reached twelve, sixteen meant that brain damage would be certain. I was desolate defiant to have suffered the plague of pregnancy only to have a mindless act of carelessness take my precious girl from me. Two more days passed the count stayed at twelve. Beautiful yellow Mary was finally removed from the incubator and placed in the zoo window. What a joy she was to look at. A head crowned with black hair. Her face had beautiful features. There was no head trauma in the birth canal she hadn't been there long enough for that to happen. The baby helper put little bows of ribbon in her beautiful long black hair. Everyone that saw her said she resembled a little Chinese baby because she was so yellow. Everyone wanted to see her. Dick was indignant. He also told all that would listen about his mother's name sake, precious Mary.

Chapter 6

They didn't know at that time that Mary would carry the results of that careless mistake with her always, but she did. Her two brothers would grow up brilliant. As a result of this negligence she would always be slow to learn, this affected her as she fought to retain comprehensive medical science that she needed as a requirement for nursing school. It did not matter how desperately she tried, she just could not master the required studies, which caused her to have to take a different route for her life.

My heart broke for my slow to learn daughter with the beautiful personality. No she was not retarded but the yellow poison had destroyed that part of her brain that would have allowed her to accomplish those things that she struggled so hard to achieve. Her lack of accomplishment in the medical field did not make us love her any less. It only caused our hearts to ache as we watched her try so hard and still not be able to master what she so longed for. One careless act took it all out of her grasp. But we are proud of our beautiful daughter and the woman she has become.

She has fought many battles but God has helped her.

Also I heard the voice of the Lord, saying: "Whom shall I send and who will go for us." Then I said, "Here am I send me."
Isaiah 6:8

My Beautiful Daughter

Chapter 1

My daughter, Mary, overcame her traumatic entry into this world. She grew up between two brothers. They had no idea what an exceptional sister they had. She caused no trouble, she took their teasing and sometimes abuse in stride. The only time she required any discipline was when she accidently used a bad word. I washed her mouth out with dish washing liquid. She was her Daddy's pride and joy. She wasn't a bikini or a two piece swim suit kind of girl. Her choice was a **"Baby Doll."**

I tried to protect her during her teenage years from trying to do things that I was sure she would certainly fail. She took these efforts as criticism. She was always a big girl from teens on.

She finished high school and wanted to become a nurse. I wanted her to try for LPN status. She could then work and get some experience with her exceptional gift of common sense. I was sure she could graduate to RN status at some point in time. Poppa wouldn't hear of it. If she is going to be a nurse she is going to be a REAL one. Off she went to pre-nursing school and did not do well. She met her husband while there.

They married and it lasted for twenty years. She had two great boys and one little brown eyed granddaughter. She brought joy to our lives. After twenty years things went into chaos. Drugs were involved. The husband, Doyle, went to pieces and threatened suicide, etc. Mary spent every bit of her grandmother's money that she left her when she died. Her grandmother had also left her some personal belongings such as crystal, silver, and all of her furniture. She had nothing left.

Doyle went to a Posh Rehab Unit in Arizona for treatment. He also required six months at a step down unit in California. Mary paid for all of it. He finally came home a changed man. Divorce was final. This was extremely stressful for my dear girl. Nobody could really help her. I prayed and tried to guide her through it.

Chapter 2

Time raced on. She finally met the man of her dreams. The match was good and they began to look for a church. They ended up helping plant a church with a very far sited pastor. The pastor had been raised in India by missionary parents. He wanted to return to the place where he grew up to see if the church seeds his parents planted had grown. This was right up Mary's ally. She went with him and has made numerous trips since to help him in their ministry.

She also established a ministry in Haiti. I am so proud of this daughter. She is the only one in the family to except this kind of a challenge. We are very proud of her and the way she is living her life. On one of her return trips from Haiti she was very ill. We took her to the Godhouse because the nausea and vomiting would not stop. They were sure she contracted something in Haiti. They sent her home thinking it would just subside on its own. The vomiting continued. We took her back to the

Godhouse insisting they do something for her, this time they admitted her. The test, x-rays, and MRI were started. They were all negative.

"We see something in the abdomen but cannot tell what it is" they said. They didn't know what to do as she lay there. Time passed but she got no better. Her attending medical Godbody was employed at the Godhouse and was an internist. There was a rule that no other Godbody of the same practice could see someone else's patient.

She lay there dying before our very eyes. She was losing weight and couldn't keep anything down for ten days. I was "falling apart" and not able to help her. I prayed and God answered. I felt him telling me to call a family friend that had grown up with our children. This person was not just a friend but a Godbody. His specialty was infectious diseases. He also was not on the Godhouse payroll. It sound like a win all the way around.

I called him and said "Mike you must come to the Godhouse. My Mary is dying! The Godbody who is following her is going to be off this week and she may not last that long. Please we are desperate!" I said with panic in my voice.

He came shortly, he looked at her records, and then came into her room. She could hardly say "hello" when he entered. Mike said, "well there is something in her belly but don't know what it is. If nothing changes by morning we are going to see what it is. Who is your surgeon?" Something positive will be done I thought. What a relief!! Praise the Lord!!!

There was no change the next morning so cutting and stitching was scheduled for the following morning. When they looked in her belly they found that the small bowel was completely obstructed. That had nothing to do with Haiti. Boy did all those Godhouse Godbodies have egg all on their faces. I had said all along forget about the fact that she was in Haiti something else is wrong and so it was. Surgery was performed and the obstruction was taken care of. My dear Mary got better and was about to go about her life as she knew it.

Chapter3

    She continues to do Gods work in Bangladesh, India and Haiti. She is still committed to her missionary work and her church. She continues to go with her pastor to Haiti once a year. Twice a year she goes and works with the Untouchables Ministry in India. These individuals are of the lower class in India. It does not matter what they do, they cannot rise above that class level. But she is faithful to the calling God has put on her heart for these people in spite of the situation they find themselves in.

    God is blessing her. I am very proud of what a smart, beautiful, wonderful and God fearing woman she has become. May god continue to bless the rest of her years.

A woman born before her time, passed on in peace.

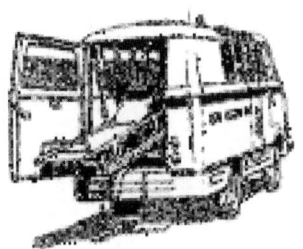

God blessed this dear lady because she kept the faith no matter what.

MR. STONE

Chapter 1

Some days are like diamonds, smooth, full of brightness, and great joy. Then there are days that are like stones, rough, dual days that have a lot to be desired. I was really having a stone type of a day when I got the call. Pop had just called from their home at the coast where they lived. He informed me that mama was in the Godhouse trying to pass a kidney stone. She was not being too successful in passing the stone when he called.

My parents didn't call often or ask for much so when they did call I was always "Johnny on the spot" to do what had to be done. Why now though? I just didn't have time for this calamity. The schedules in the Cutting and Stitching Shop had been unreal lately. Everyone was working from the time they can until they couldn't any longer. There was just no way to catch up. There was an unfounded rumor that an emergency head opening had been on the schedule for three days. I hadn't checked but it was probably true. I didn't see how I could take off now, but I must. I bade farewell to the Shop promising to be back as soon as possible. The four hour drive to the coast seemed like eight. I thought I would never get there. I left at daybreak, arrived before lunch to find Mama in a really bad state.

Chapter 2

As I sat with Mama I was very concerned about how the stone was acting. It seemed that the stone had passed from the kidney down the ureter tube and was lodged about six inches from the bladder. From time to time old Mr. Stone would change positions, block the ureter, back urine up into the kidney and send Mama's blood pressure plummeting, putting her in shock. She was also running a fever. Damn, something had to be done, and now! I was informed that a special kidney Godbody was coming over at about six p.m. for a consultation.

That was good, I thought but in the meantime we are going to try and turn that rock into a rolling stone. Once it passed into the bladder they would be home free. On came the fluids, what a better way to make the stone roll. I made Mama drink six ounces of something every hour on the hour. Mama was tough and willing to drink what I offered her. She did great until five o'clock. Then she started gaging on everything I offered. Neither the nurses nor I could think of anything else to give her to drink, the choice was limited because she was a severe diabetic.

Chapter 3

The kidney Godbody arrived. He sent for a stretcher for Mama to take her to the Cutting-Stitching Shop. "What in heaven's name is he going to do?" I asked almost in a screaming voice. I was informed by the poison-passer that he was going to try and get the stone. "This can't be," I cried.

I knew this procedure called for general body poison that has to be on an empty stomach. Nobody had told us that this was going to be done. We had already stuffed her full of various and sundry food and solutions. There was no preparation. I could hardly contain my rage as they wheeled her away. I knew that Mama mustn't know the possible fate that she was facing at that moment. I knew what might take place. I had never been in such a damnable situation. My choices were to show my ass and stop the whole show or take the chance that Mama would drown in her own vomit as she was put to sleep. This is totally unacceptable I fumed inside myself. It would never have happened in my shop. The procedure could have waited for a safer time. They didn't because it was not convenient for the consulting Godbody. I was in a mental kaleidoscope, unable to make a decision.

The procedure started. My agony continued four long endless hours. I made a promise that as sure as there was a God in heaven that I would never let this happen again. Finally they told me that Mama was in the wake up room but that the stone was still stuck. I made a decision then and there that come morning this Godhouse would be just a reflection in the rear view mirror of an ambulance. I was taking Mama to my Godhouse where she would at least be safe.

Chapter 4

Morning dawned and there was no change in Mama's status. I began making preparation to make Mama mobile. I was getting her out of this place. The personal Godbody was very upset at the whole situation but mostly because I was moving her from his clutches. He said, "Oh if I had just known what was happening last night, I would have NEVER subjected your mother to that risk."

Uh, huh and my Aunt Effie plays for the Brooklyn Dodgers I thought. I was sure the only thing he was sorry for was the fact that he was losing the revenue that my Moms' stone was generating for him. I kept these thoughts to myself. I just smiled and said, "please give me what I need to make this move, if you will, and pray that we make it."

Chapter 5

In those days ambulance service consisted of transfer, no treatment. I armed myself with a syringe of Epinephrine, a small tank of O_2 and a prayer for a fast driver. The ambulance arrived, we loaded Mama in, and was ready for our trip of what would normally be four hours. But hopefully on this day it would be a lot faster than when I came.

"Careful, don't rock the boat, we are not ready for a rolling stone at this point," I joked with the driver. I was trying desperately not to let Mama see that I was petrified. I knew that they were in some hard place, careful but fast. I knew that if Mama was left in this limited service Godhouse they would surely kill her. They had tried that last night doing the surgery on a full stomach. On the other hand there was a very good chance that Mr. Stone could decide to change his position, block the urine path and cause her blood pressure to bottom out and yes, death could come to visit her as they sped down the highway.

I was certain that they must take the chance. I briefed the driver and his co-pilot as to the gravity of the situation. They assured me that the pedal would be on the medal and the siren open. We were off! I thought my heart would literally explode. I tried not to take her blood pressure to often but I had to occupy my mind with something. I sat beside Mama where I could see the speedometer while I was pondering the situation. I could not believe my eyes it was a constant ninety, ninety-five and one hundred miles an hour. I didn't know which aspect of the situation scared me the most, Mama going into shock or the speed at which we were traveling.

I will surely have a stroke if I don't get a hold of myself, I thought. I know, I will concentrate on swimming, which will help me calm down. I commanded my brain to start thinking. Lord, how I love swimming. I could do some fine synchronized swimming strokes just like the famous Ester

Williams. I was deep in thought when Mama interrupted with the question, "what time is it?" I came back to reality and replied, "9:30." "Where are we?" was the next question. "We are in Lucedale," I replied to her. "Humph, I could have made it faster in my little ole Dodge!" she grumbled I ascertained that they were sixty miles down the road and they had departed the Godhouse at exactly nine o'clock. I laughed to myself because I knew her car couldn't begin to go as fast as we were going. I just kept smiling as looking into her loving face.

Chapter 6

I only remember the rest of the trip in bits and pieces. I thought if migraines were really brought on by stress I would certainly have a doozy of one today. The only thing in this day was stress. I still recall the indescribable joy and the overwhelming feeling of relief when Mama was unloaded in the emergency room of my very own Godhouse. I sighed with relief knowing now she would be taken care of properly.

Two days passed and the stone had not moved so they did abdominal surgery. She was taken home two days later. She had gotten an infection and since my husband stayed there with her they trained him on how to change the dressing. He helped nurse her back to health.

They got very close in those days. She would tell everyone that would listen to her that nurses think they know everything. Then she would look at Dick with a smile on her face and twinkle in her eye and say, "he's my main stay." When she completely recovered, she went back to her house on the coast. How thankful we were for her full recovery.

What a delightful soul!!

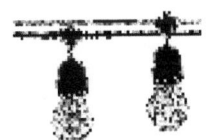

She lived with a perfect faith in God.

AN EXCEPTIONAL WOMAN

Chapter1

My in-laws were Italian. They very much followed the Italian ways especially in the naming of their children. The first son was named after their father, the first daughter named after the father's mother, and the third child can be named by the child's mother. They had five grandchildren and two were born on my father-in-law's birthday. We did this with our children as generations had done before us. What stories they told about how it was in the day. I would find myself almost in tears with laughter. The ones I recall today still make me laugh.

My mother-in-law had one of her own traditions. She would crochet each grandchild a red toboggan by the time they were three years old. I still have the ones she made for our three children. They are just the cutest. One day I will pass them on but right now I will treasure them and keep them safe until that time comes.

    She was a wonderfully bright person. She had a great sense of humor. I can still see her trim body, never over one hundred and thirty five pounds. Her contagious smile would make the room lighten up. She had beautiful gray hair by the age of fifty that eventually turned snow white. She was into taking care of herself; therefore she never drank or smoked. It also might have had something to do with the fact that she was a devout Catholic. She attended a church just two blocks from her house. She walked most of the time. I never asked her but I figured it was because it was good exercise. She also said that some days she changed her cloths up to five times. Her changing pattern, when she got up early she got dressed went to kitchen to drink coffee, then she would change to go to church, when she got home from church she would change to get diner, if she was going to the spa she would have to change again, when she got back from the spa she changed again, the last change would be if she was going to church again. Wow, five times in one day, she kept herself busy those days just changing her cloths.

Boy could she cook. I can still see the homemade noodles hanging all over the house while they dried. It makes my mouth water for their delicious taste as I think of them even to this day and it has been many years since I have had that delicious taste to cross my lips. She did not neglect her house work either. She was an avid housekeeper. I don't know how she did everything she did.

Chapter 2

It was extremely tough buying her presents. She was very frugal and did not want money spent on flowers, even though she really enjoyed them. She said it was a waste of money, she could grow them. At Christmas she even said "I don't need that. You keep it. You could get better use of it than I can." It didn't matter what it was. What a challenge but I was determined to find something I could get her that she would like. I was on the hunt for the perfect gift. One day while we were visiting I thought I would snoop in the bathroom to see if I could discover a hidden secret I yet did not know about. There it was, staring me right in the face: cosmetics. I took note of the special brand she used and patted myself on the back as I waited for the next special occasion. When it arrived I presented her with the cosmetics I noticed she was low on and just smiled. That was the beginning of her keeping the gifts I gave. Yes, I was pleased with my accomplishment.

She was plagued with bad deformities of arthritis, especially in her hands. She routinely went to a local spa and sat in the whirlpool. She said they ask me "Mrs. Gloriso do you have children?" "Oh yes I have a son who is fifty." She was talking about my husband Dick, her baby. She said "I don't even tell them about Francis who is ten years older than Dick". She had a couple favorite saying. One was, "I am not getting older. My clothes are what's getting older". The other one, "I've been married all of my life and I've been working since I was born." She had to help take care of her siblings since she was the oldest of seven.

Chapter 3

At the age of seventy five she had to have back surgery. I went to New Orleans to stay with her for a week after she came home from the hospital. After she was home, she began to vomit. There was no relief even at night it continued all night long. We discovered she was highly allergic to anything called anesthesia. She survived, which we were thankful for.

When she got older it was time for her to have cataract surgery. Oh boy I thought. I sent Dick to New Orleans this time to see about her. Surgery went well so Dick was able to take her home. Then the vomiting started and continued through the night. Dick called me very concerned about his mother. In panic he said to me "mother is confused, her balance is not good and I have to take her to the bathroom." My first thought was stroke. "Is she weak on one side?" I asked. "No just generalized weakness and confusion. She couldn't even find her way around the house" he replied. "Then take her back to the surgeon" I advised. He did. They assessed her as being dehydrated and gave her I.V. fluids unfortunately, it didn't help a lot. Dick called again even more alarmed "mother is not getting any better" he said in a panic. "Take her to her family doctor," I instructed him.

Her family doctor, Dr. Long, assessed her, and looked at her history and noticed her allergy to anesthetic. He figured out she was having a reaction to the anesthetic she was given for her surgery. He gave her an IV and continued a routine spectrum of vitamins and electrolytes. Mother woke up feeling better. When she told her story, she said, I vomited so much all my electric light went out. We all laughed at her humor even in this time of fright. What a woman that mother-in law of mine!

I was furious that the other doctor did not catch her allergy to the anesthetic. He had it all right there in her records. I tried not to stew on that for long. We were just very thankful that Dr. Long was able to figure it out and get her on the road to recovery.

God is good all the time even when we don't know what else to do. He sends someone to help. Thanks to Dr. Long for being that person for us at that time.

Life is filled
with battles to
win or lose.
He won!!

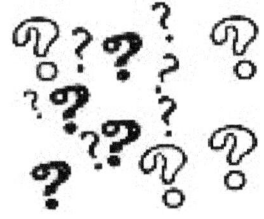

When we are ready to give up

God provides with the perfect

answer.

THE MYSTERY

Chapter 1

Dick was an internist nightmare. He was first generation Italian, thirty pounds overweight, high blood pressure since he was twenty and smoked like a chimney in winter. He ate only things that he liked; for example red meat, salt on everything, bread and butter, and lots of sweets. His favorite was Hersey Chocolate bars which he sat on, to help soften them, so they could be eaten easier. He liquefied his ice cream by zapping it in the microwave. He also routinely used five spoons of sugar in his coffee. He liked his orange juice that way and drank coke instead of water. No surprise that he suffered from occasional gout attacks because of his crazy diet along with his other ailments. He was a complainer; my legs hurt, I have a headache, I have indigestion, and the beat went on. There was always something wrong. He had a very low pain threshold. He was also the most non-physical person I have ever known, except for his best buddy Bob. Instead of "couch potatoes" I call them "laz-e-boy turnips" only moving from the loungers for absolute necessities. I do believe that they would drive to the bathroom if they could get the car in the house! Dick's philosophy regarding any type of exercise was that "the good Lord gave your old heart so many ticks" if you used them up too fast, too bad. That is why so many people have heart attacks. So he felt slowing down physical activities would not use those ticks up as quickly. There seems to be some credence to his way of thinking, look at those deaths during strenuous exercise. Also a friend of ours, who we will call Bill, watched his diet, not a pound overweight, didn't smoke, drank in moderation, and exercised regularly, ended up having a triple heart by-pass. Bill told me that every time he woke up in the recovery room from his by-pass he thought about Dick's saying that a person only has so many ticks. Of course me being a nurse and Dick's wife believe that the answer to this riddle is that Dick and Bob are both laid back. They don't give a shit if the sun doesn't shine, real type B personalities. While Bill is a type A personality, do right, push hard, can't make a mistake, he set very high standard for himself. Well, that is my philosophy of the men. Obviously, I had very little patience with Dick or his parade of pain, most of which, in my mind, he brought on himself. However, this episode would teach me to appreciate him in a way I hadn't in the thirty years we had been together.

Chapter 2

This particular Friday in April of 1982 was a very special day for Dick. He was going to see his favorite Internist for his annual physical. "I suppose you have done the usual," I asked him as he came popping into the kitchen grinning.

"Yep, no chocolate, no sugar, no salt, no ice cream for a whole week, I can't wait to get this over with. Want some steak tonight?" he asked with an even bigger grin on his face. I think he already tasted it in his mind.

"I guess," I answered. I knew there was no need to argue with him. All the health food arguments had been used up years ago.

"I came through the check up with flying colors," he announced when he arrived home. "But I did get a new prescription for this gout."

I guess the new prescription was to justify the three hundred and fifty dollars he charged him to tell him he was in good shape considering the circumstances. I thought as I watched Dick fix his favorite meal, filet, French fries, and French bread with lots of butter. How does he get away with it, I wondered as I cut up broccoli to eat with the small steak he had cooked for me. After we finished eating Dick flopped down in his laz-e-boy and began to complain about how his toe hurt. I figured he was anxious to try out his new pills. I gave him two pills with his coke. He swallowed them and leaned back to continue his rest for the evening.

 The next evening when he returned home from playing bridge with his cronies of thirty years, he was scowling and red faced he said, "Honey, I have a terrible headache and my toe is still not feeling any better. Please find my medicine."

 I got his medicine for his gout along with Bufferin for his headache. He took those and shortly after we were headed to bed. The nighttime brought a little fever, general aches and pains, more Bufferin compulsory fluids and lots of tender loving care from me. Sunday passed with little change. The flu had come to visit or so we thought.

Chapter 3

He screamed as we woke on Monday morning, "I can hardly move my arm, and I can't stand on my left foot." His face reflected his horror and disbelief as he found his left side didn't work.

Oh my God, a stroke I thought. Well, I wasn't really surprised, but shocked anyway. I've warned him a thousand times about fat, salt and his laziness. But now was not the time to remind him of any of that. I stepped into action and called his internist. After I relayed his symptoms, the doctor agreed and wanted me to bring him immediately to the Catholic Godhouse. I did just that. When the internist arrived he evaluated the situation and verified the stroke diagnosis.

"Put Dick in bed immediately," he ordered and started the barrage of studies that are subjected to on every Godhouse admission. Dick seemed to be in shock as his veins were stuck for blood, x-rays taken, and the EKG's were run. I was madder than hell, wondering why he didn't take better care of his self. The afternoon brought negative results from all the tests and weakness in Dick's other arm and leg set in. Oh no, wrong diagnosis, definitely not a stoke. Consultation was sought from the second Godbody, a Neurologist. He agreed it wasn't a stroke, nor is it a neurological deficit.

"What is it?" I asked almost in a scream of panic. "Could it be his gout medicine? That is the only thing he has done different."

"No, I doubt it," he said as he made his exit. I guess he thought he had earned his five hundred dollars, because that was all he said as he left. No more words of help or comfort. Well, I thought, he did tell us what it wasn't.

Chapter 4

Next in the Godbody parade was a neurosurgeon, to rule out brain tumor. Bull shit I thought, it is inconceivable that Dick came from a clean bill of health on Friday to paralysis from a brain tumor on Wednesday. It just doesn't work that way. The neurosurgeon doctor ordered more tests and studies. He had enough blood drawn by now to stain the ocean, enough x-rays to cause radiation, not to mention sterility. They had found nothing!! Not a stroke or a brain tumor, but what is going on? We didn't see the neurosurgeon again but we did see his bill.

My heart was heavy, frustration level high, and tears flowed as I strived to comfort my helpless husband. All his joints were red and swollen, he had bilateral foot drop, he couldn't walk, sit or turn himself in bed. He was in excruciating pain. He said "even my hair hurts." He screamed when he was touched. Several nurses left his room crying because they could not help him. He was requiring Demerol and Valium every two to three hours. In my mind I had concluded that he would surely die and do so an addict.

Chapter 5

Due to his swollen, red joints, Godbody number four, a female rheumatologist arrived upon the scene. She poked, listened, looked and decided that Dick had a rare liver disease caused by chronic alcohol intake.

"I am the drinker in the family, not Dick," I informed her, "unless coke classic counts. Could the new medication that they gave him for gout cause this?" I asked with frustration in my voice.

"How long since he stopped drinking?" she asked. She was very persistent. **"Maybe he only drank wine or beer?"** By this time she was sitting on a chair near the bed with his chart in her lap and pen poised ready to write it all down. I could not help but notice her typical Asian features contrasted sharply against her white lab coat. "Oh dear," she purred, "unless you are honest with me I cannot help you."

"That's enough," I said in a very loud voice. She is accusing us of lying I thought rising from the lumpy day bed where I had spent the last six nights. I neared her and continued, "The man doesn't, nor has he ever drank alcohol, he doesn't like it. Furthermore, if you put in the records that he does drink, you will see us in court." I was fuming, "can't you see you're barking up the wrong tree?"

    The Rheumatologist slammed the chart closed and rose to leave the room. I thought this helped her get the point. I was trembling as I sat back on the day bed. She seemed to read my mind, if she had a tail it would have been between her legs as she slunk out the door. I didn't give her another thought until I received the seven hundred and fifty dollar bill that reminded me of her incompetent, unpleasant intrusion.

Chapter 6

The next player in this nightmare is Godbody number five, a plastic surgeon. He wants to biopsy Dick's foot. Well, why not, I thought. We are now grasping at straws. I assumed that this minor procedure would be done in Dick's room for his comfort, such things are done every day in the doctor's office. I was soooooooooo wrong this time. He was hauled off, screaming all the way to the operating room. Why? I wondered. Then the reason hit me. Of course, this brought more revenue in for the Godbody and the Godhouse, "a surgical procedure!" This too proved fruitless. All tests were negative. Anyone reading the test results in Dick's chart would have assumed that he was a healthy man. How shocking to see this frozen shell of a man screaming in agony, lying helpless, bed ridden, slowly becoming addicted to the pain killing Demerol.

Time crept by. Days and nights seemed to melt together. He was surely dying, shots, pills, and all the efforts was to no avail. There is one more Godbody we haven't tried, mine, I thought. He had performed a miracle for me when he diagnosed my Rocky Mountain Spotted Fever, which four others missed. My God, if he could just do a repeat performance for poor Dick, I would be grateful. After working through the Godbody protocol regarding having two internists on the same case, Godbody number six arrived. He was my personal Godbody. He stood well over six feet tall, had big brown eyes, a handsome figure of a man but today he was grumpy. He clearly resented the position I had put him in by insisting that he see Dick. He did his usual thorough things: poked, prodded, felt listened, looked and didn't talk much. He didn't tell us what he thought was wrong. I knew better than to ask. He wrote his recommendations in the chart and he was off. We found out later when we obtained Dick's' records that they were not followed. He was the only one who had solved this mystery, but his instructions were not even followed. So Dick still did not get any better.

Chapter 7

Easter came and went, we prayed, Dick screamed. No hope left, we had run the gamut of Godbodies. It had occurred to me several times that Dick looked like one big "gout" from head to toe. I had mentioned this to several of the Godbodies, matter of fact, I had asked all five of the doctors could it be the new gout medicine he was given. They had shrugged it off in their usual "nurses are smart asses" manner. Well, this smart ass just had to get my hands on the PDR, laughingly called a Physician Desk Reference on drugs. I asked one of the more compassionate nurses it there was one at the desk. She brought it to me. I looked under **Benimid.** There I found Dick's condition perfectly described, red, swollen joints, foot drop, and excruciating pain. He was in the thrones of a violent drug reaction! We had done everything the PDR said not to do when taking this drug. Aspirin or any of its products were not to be taken in conjunction with this medication, according to the book. I was astounded!!! If just one of those high and mighty bastards had bothered to use their PDR what a different story this would have been.

My heart was pounding against my chest, because I was furious. I am sure blue fire was sparking from my eyes. Oh the urge to kill, it was a good thing that there wasn't a Godbody in site. I told Dick what I found. I watched life spring back into his eyes. I said, "I'll be back," and I left the room to take care of business. Taking control myself, I drove to my office, laid the PDR on the copier and ran five copies. I then took a red pen and underlined all of Dick's symptoms and wrote the name of all our Godbodies at the top and headed back to the Godhouse. I returned to that horrific room once more to collect Dick.

"Honey, take me home before these SOB's finish killing me," Dick said as he looked at me with tears in his pleading brown eyes. I was looking into the eyes of my husband who was pathetic and permanently damaged.

"Will you stop at the nurse's station," I asked the aide that was pushing the wheel chair Dick was in.

"Sure," was her replied and stopped as we arrived.

"Will you see that these get to the people whose names are on them?" I asked as I handed the copies I had made to the nurse that loaned me the PDR. She looked confused just for a second then a smile like the Florida sunshine split her face.

"It'll be my pleasure," she replied, "sister smart ass." I chuckled and Dick smiled for the first time in twenty-two days.

Upon arriving home I stopped all gout medication. He gradually began to improve, within a week he was able to walk. In the next two to three weeks he was getting back to his normal self. I had hoped this would help learn a lesson about a healthier lifestyle but I was wrong. He continued in the unhealthy lifestyle that he was accustomed to. Oh what a man.

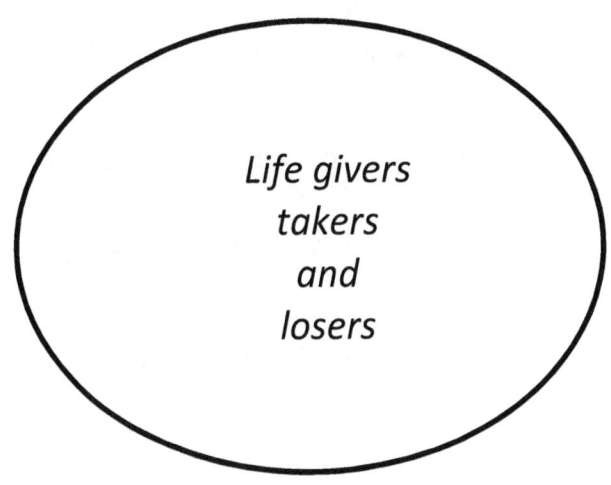

*Life givers
takers
and
losers*

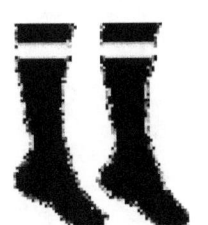

Life without God is utter darkness. God delivered them from alcohol but they did not become God people.

LIFE STOCKINGS

Chapter 1

What would we do without dear friends? Ones that we could do fun and not so fun things with. We had such friends, Bill and Patsy. We had been friends for many years. Bill was medium built, big brown eyes, brown hair and an olive complexion. His wife was much the same. But they both had a big downfall, and that was drinking. It wasn't just one or two drinks, too many times it was the falling down flat on their face kind of problem. To the point many nights we had to take them home. None the less we enjoyed having them come over and play bridge. Bill even nicknamed my husband, Dick, Pal. We all had a great time playing then we would drive them home when it was merited.

When we would go places I tried to avoid bridge with Patsy if I could because of her drinking problem. I remember one time very vividly. We were at a bridge tournament in Natchez, the guys had gone for the masters. I had no other choice but to go with Patsy. Keep in mind it is not her that I do not like, it is all the drinking. In a different room there were ten to fifteen side tables we signed up to play at one of those side games. I noticed the drinks kept coming. I began to count, she had fourteen total. I could not believe it. Maybe I should have been thankful for those considering we did end up in second place. Yeah us!!! I couldn't help but think how we might have been first had she not been drinking OR was that how we ended up second. What a night that was.

Chapter 2

I'm not quite sure when but at some time during our friendship, our friends stopped the drinking. There was no explanation they just did. They did it cold turkey. That was a great thing for them.

A few years had passed and Bill ended up in the hospital for a vascular bypass. The procedure was called, a femoral-bypass to his left leg. It was a fairly simple surgery. It was done on a Thursday. We went to the hospital to see him on Friday on our way out of town to the coast. He was sitting up in bed, cheerful and talking. We visited for a while and everything seemed to be going very good for him. As we left he bid us farewell and to have a good time.

I was bothered as I walked to the car about the fact Bill was not wearing the anti-embolism hose. I knew these were routine for most types of surgery and especially for any type of vascular procedure he just underwent. They helped the circulation of the blood so blood clots didn't form. I was in hopes that I just didn't notice them on him. When we got into the car I asked my husband if he noticed if Bill was wearing the anti-embolism hose. He confirmed my great fear that he was not. My heart was heavy, because I knew blood clots could end with bad results. We drove on to the coast but I could not get the fact that Bill did not have anti-embolism stockings on, out of my mind. I should have said something I kept telling myself. I know those sock can help save lives, even though people don't like wearing them at times. It was not the most pleasant trip I had ever made to the coast, it also seemed to last longer than a couple of days. I was anxious to hear how Bill was doing. I prayed he was doing well.

Chapter 3

What a shock we had when we returned home on Sunday. Bill had died from an embolism. I know that an embolism is caused by obstruction of an artery, typically by a clot of blood or air bubble. I deeply regretted not questioning the fact that he was not wearing the stockings on Friday. I was filled with guilt and will always regret not speaking up. But for now I knew I just needed to shake myself so I could be of help to Patsy. She was in shock and needed any help I could grant.

Patsy was beside herself trying to get all the details of the funeral in order. They did not belong to a church so they had no pastor to help. She had asked my husband to say a few words. Dick really had no idea what to say but how could he say no. The service was going to be at the funeral home. Patsy had said it was going to be casual. As the other final plans were being made, Dick was on his mission of finding something to say. He started looking in the

Bible for an easy scripture to read. He didn't know where to begin. He was a Catholic, he didn't attend mass, so he was not familiar with the Bible. That did not stop him. He put himself to the task and came up with an acceptable presentation. He would do anything for his dear friend that he would greatly miss.

Chapter 4

The day of the funeral we dressed painfully slow and casual according to what Patsy had said. Dick drove extra sluggishly that day. He was in no big hurry to tell his good friend goodbye for the last time. As we entered the chapel we were stunned at the great crowd of suits, ties and dresses. There stood me in my slacks and Dick in his short sleeve shirt and no tie. We took only a moment to survey the surroundings then proceeded in. I spied Patsy and took a seat next to her.

We arrived early. As we sat lost in our grief staring into space the chapel director taped on Patsy shoulder. "What music would you liked played" he asked in his soft voice. She was shocked and puzzled at the question. Matter of fact so was I. I thought that should have already been taken care of, not here at the last minute. Since they did not attend church and she was uncertain as to what to tell him. He questioned her again "Is there a song you would like or does he have a favorite one?" After thinking for another moment she said "Sentimental Journey". As the people came and went Sentimental Journey played.

    I know that is not the typical kind of song for that occasion but the words did seem to fit.

    "Gonna take a sentimental journey

    Gonna set my heart at ease

    Gonna make a sentimental journey

    To renew old memories

    Got my bag, got my reservation

    Spent each dime I could afford

    Like a child in wild anticipation

    Long to hear that 'all aboard'

    Seven, that's the time to leave, at seven

    I'll be waitin' in heaven

    Countin' every mile of railroad track

    That takes me back...

    Seven, that's the time we leave, at seven

    I'll be waitin' up in heaven

    Countin' every mile of railroad track

That takes me back

Never thought my heart could be so 'yearny'

Why did I decide to roam?

Gotta take that sentimental journey

Sentimental journey home

Bill was on his last journey. One at this present time we cannot follow but someday we all will take that journey. I sat there next to my dear friend and prayed that God would comfort her and help her through this time of grief.

"Good-bye dear friend" I said in my mind as I passed by and took my last gaze upon his face. Patsy and I walked hand in hand out of the chapel after she said her last good-bye. We face our own journey without this dear friend and husband to walk alongside us now.

Life stockings have taught me a valuable lesson. I determined to always speak up when I think it could help save a person's life. God give me the courage to speak up for others.

Do you know where your balance is?

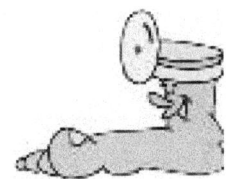

God gave everything a great purpose and our toe serves as our balance.

HONORABLE TOE

Chapter 1

It was a typical morning and I was getting ready to start my day. I lazily went to the kitchen to get breakfast before going to work. I went to the refrigerator to get milk for my cereal. I saw that the milk man had been at the house earlier and left fresh milk which I was glad. I reached in grabbed the glass bottle of milk it was slippery and slipped right out of my hand. It shattered as it hit the floor. I could not believe I had done that, I did not have time for such a mess this morning I thought to myself. When I looked down, there was blood everywhere. My right big toe had been cut.

I wrapped It the best I could then quickly called the Operating Room to schedule an appointment to have repairs made to the toe. I arrived at the OR and they went to work on repairing the toe. They fixed the tendon then put the toe in a cast. While they worked I was thinking since I was already at the hospital I might as well go on to work after they finished. I was advised to go home after they put the cast on but I had already decided I would stay and work. I hobbled around with that cast on for three weeks, it was the most uncomfortable thing. At the end of the three weeks I was rejoicing with the thoughts of the cast finally coming off. I was in for a great big surprise, they took off the cast and the toe went flop. The repair had not worked!! The repair had to be done all over again. I could not believe it.

Chapter 2

I had a trip planned for San Diego that I just could not cancel. I had to have the repair when I returned. I packed my bags and off I flew, messed up toe and all. It was very hard to walk when your big toe is injured, but try putting on dress shoes and trying to act like nothing was wrong. That is a chore. I could only wear flats and opened toes. It was February and cold but I did what I needed to do. I held the toe up and slid it in my shoe. I was very proud of myself I only fell three times. The pain was awful but I kept going.

Chapter 3

Upon my return home I prepared for the repair that needed to be done to my toe. To the hospital I trusted this time the repair would be correct and I could get on with my life. A spinal had to be done when they did the repair. This time they put on a boot that went up to my knee. The strangest thing happened. I began to have pain but it was not at point of the repair in the toe, it was in the back of my leg. I complained but no one was taking note. I did not keep quiet I kept on complaining, in spite of the fact they told me that could not be.

I finally convinced an intern that there was a problem with the back of my leg. He informed me that the boot was not to be taken off. But I insisted that he look. He gave in, against the wishes of the regular doctor, and took the boot off to see what was happening. When he removed it he found blood blisters on the back of my leg. The blisters were where the nurse was holding my leg while they were putting on the cast on my toe. They took the boot off but I had to have the dressing changed every day.

I had asked the doctor if he could stop by the hospital on his way to his office to change the dressing but he would not. I could not drive so it was very inconvenient for me to find a ride every day. I could make the room ready and it would have taken him only a few minutes to do the dressing. He was very arrogant and would not even consider helping me out. I did go to his office and get the dressing changed. The whole idea that he was not willing to do a service that was within reason to me was unthinkable. I sued him not for what happened but the attitude he had about not being considerate to his patient.

Beware of strangers eating your chips.

God made all creatures big and small.

THE UNWANTED GUEST

Chapter 1

Yippee, yippee, and yahoo, I yelled to myself as I flew down highway nineteen toward Neshoba County. The red hills slipped by me. What a beautiful sight. Lord, how I love these hills, I thought as I drove. Sometimes I think I am like Scarlett O'Hara and Tara in "Gone With the Wind." "I get my strength from these hills" they would say. If I am away too long I get soul-sick. To me the hills, are a living breathing entity; they are fertile, beautiful and permanent. They contain my roots and the dirt covers the remains of the most important person in my life, my grandmother.

She was uneducated but Solomon would say she was wise. She had an innate knowledge of the right and wrong of things. She never wavered from them. Bless her, I thought. I would have never made it through my early childhood years without her. I have got to go and see about her grave for the hundredth time I thought. But there is no hurry. I know she understands.

My grandmother's face often comes before me with her twinkly blue eyes. She always wore a bonnet that matched her apron. The bonnet covered her silver grey hair which was worn in a bun at the nape of her neck. Her apron always had a pocket that carried her small silver snuff box. I was always fascinated by the decorum and the dignity that she lent to this usually disgusting habit. Her snuff box had a tiny spoon attached to the lid. She would measure the precise amount of snuff, place it just off-center in her lower lip and that was the last you saw of it. I was one of the few people ever to see her indulge in this little habit. It was the only sin that kept her out of the church. I know in my bones, if there is a heaven, she is in it. Even now sometimes when I am troubled I can feel her presence, can hear her council and see her smile of encouragement.

"Well, Granny, I hope you can see me now, looking forward to a real country weekend." As I crossed the Neshoba County line the stress, worry and aggravation of the weeks past just washed away by the pure, fresh clean air. What a great weekend I was sure to have.

Chapter 2

I headed for a house that I had built for my mother. She never lived in it and I was stuck with it. The furnishings and the lake-location are the only things that reflect any part of me. But it is comfortable and serves my purpose. Oh, how wonderful not to have a schedule, no telephone obligations, and not to be around people unless I decided I wanted to be, freedom from the city for a real country weekend. I sat and thought of all the things I could do, burrow in and read a good book, putter around the lake, maybe even fish. I could even go exploring the back fifteen acres which the house sat on. I might even plant those gladiola bulbs I have had for a while.

I might visit my older brother Bill. We needed to start planning next year's garden anyway. He loved to talk about the garden. But I knew that when it came time to plant I would be the one to head the crew. I was always the one getting the hard work done. No matter, I loved to see growing things in progress, knowing I would enjoy the finished produce.

Maybe I'll pay a visit to my cousin Maureen. She always kept me up on all the country family happenings and has a real zeal for life. Time spent with her is always refreshing. Back to the basic time of childhood, the choices of topics were always mind clearing and thought renewing.

Around dark I arrived at my little house. It was five miles from nowhere. I had no inkling that this was going to be a night of reckoning. I unloaded the car, clothes that I had taken home and washed and of course some of my favorite things to eat, Nutty-Buddy candy bars, Rice Crispies and whole milk for my coffee. I unpacked my clothes making sure everything was ready for the days ahead. Then I ate a Nutty-Buddy bar and settled down with the latest Lawrence Sanders' novel. I was ready for a great night.

Chapter 3

All the freedom exultation caused my eyes to droop around ten o'clock. I locked up and by eleven I was in a dreamless sleep. I never dream. I stopped telling anybody this because it is a known fact in the medical world only the hopelessly insane never dream! So be it; another exception to the rule.

Two o'clock in the morning --- **click, clickety**, was the sound coming from the kitchen. My eyes flew open and I bolted upright in my bed. Something or someone was in the house! I eased my feet to the floor, slid the dresser drawer open, and got my .38 pistol. **Click, clickety, scratch**. My heart was beating like a drum against my chest wall. My shaking hand clenched the pistol. My mind screamed and I was in panic mode. I had been warned many times not to come up here alone. But I did not listen! Was tonight going to be the night I wished I had taken my family and friends advice? Thoughts along with reason kept racing through my head. Call somebody!!! I could be dead before they got here. Run!! Where? I couldn't turn my back on whatever is in that back room. **Click, clickety, scratch**, that noise just would not stop. I have to see what it is. I crept down the hall mustering up every ounce of courage I possessed. I got to the door of the kitchen, took a deep breath, stuck my left hand inside the door jam and flipped the light switch.

The light came on. My head swam, my eyes refused to focus for a split second. Then I saw the biggest raccoon I could have ever imagined. In my shock and amazement he appeared to be at least ten feet tall. He was sitting on the table with an opened bag of chips eating. "Damn you," I yelled. "I'll just shoot your ass." Phsitt, phsitt, the monster hissed, bearing his upper teeth. They looked like they might be a foot long.

In my mind I was still trying to figure out what to do. What if I miss my shot and it just makes him madder? I could see him leaping at my face, tearing into my jugular vein. "Mary Mother of God, what do

I do?" I prayed. "Get out of here," I screamed to the beast.

"Phsitt, phsitt" was his reply to my screaming. I'd just have to shoot, my hands shook as I raised the gun. If I hit him in the head he'd just bleed all over my carpet, if I wounded him he would surely attack. While all these things raced through my mind he gave a final phsitt, turned and went out the way he'd come in, which was by the window air conditioning unit in the other bedroom.

I returned to my bed and sat there for a second trembling. Then I flew to examine the window. Sure enough, the extenders for the air conditioner had rotted and the raccoon had pushed through. I frantically looked around for something to plug the hole. I did not want any more unwelcomed guess this night or at any time matter of fact. I packed a pillow on one side, found a plastic trash can that exactly fit the other side and stuffed it in there. As I gave the final shove I thought, I'll never get back to sleep but I made myself walk back down the hall to my bed. I laid my pistol on top of the nightstand because it had taken too long to get it out of the dresser door and if I had another emergency I did not want to waste not even a split second. I will leave it right here in reach and patted my faithful companion. My dreamless sleep finally came to my weary body.

    A **crackle, crackle** sound reached my ears again. I jerked to a sitting position and opened my tired eyes to see it was only four a.m. Now what! Again I was filled with panic. That raccoon could not possibly have gotten back in. **Crackle! Crackle!** It was coming from the kitchen, again. Gun in hand, I slowly moved in that direction. I drew courage from the fact that I had just executed this routine. Even my heart and hands were behaving a little better. So I continued my walk down the hall toward the kitchen.

    I flipped on the kitchen light and sure enough, Mr. Raccoon was back. This time he was sitting astride my microwave enjoying my chips. Seriously I thought. **Crackle, crackle** came the sound from the package. Whoosh, relief, at the same time some fear returned like an echo. As my mind repeated the same thoughts, shoot, miss, jugular. "What are you doing?" I screamed. As if he was going to answer.

Phsitt, phsitt. He eyed me with a warning look. Not that he was afraid of me or my gun. He was in full control, the catbird seat I like to call it. Chips were sticking out from his teeth. I opened the sliding glass door, laid the gun on the counter and grabbed a broom from the closet. Maybe I can beat him off I thought if he attacked. I made a sweeping motion toward him in hoped he would run out the door.

"Go! Get out of here! Get, phsitt!" I yelled I ventured a little closer, waving the broom. Plunk he jumped to the floor. I made a sweeping mothing toward the door. With a final **'phsitt'** he whirled and went down the hall back into a bedroom. Not what I had anticipated but I slammed the door to the bedroom. "I'll just leave your butt there. Come daylight I'll get Bill to help me dispose of you for good." I said feeling proud of myself.

Chapter 4

Now it was four-thirty. I felt like I had had no sleep. I have got to try and get some sleep I told myself as I stretched out on the bed, still shaky. I closed my eyes then they popped wide open. Raccoon can open things, I remembered. Momma made a pet out of one when I was only eight. One day when we came home from town we found he had taken the top off of a jar of syrup. He was sitting on the table eating it with his paws. Syrup was on everything. The whole house was a sticky mess. He had apparently dunked his paws, licked, then walked around more than one time. We were cleaning up syrup for over a week. We thought we would never get this mess cleaned up. Yes, they can open things and this has already been proven. What if he opened the cotton-picking door! With this in mind I jumped out of bed and barricaded that bedroom door with the dresser and chest of drawers. Now maybe I can get some much needed rest.

When I woke from the little sleep I was able to get, the night horrors came rushing back in on me or was it a dream. Did I finally have a dream? No! I wished that was all it was but the dresser and chest were still against the door. Maybe I had done that in my sleep I reasoned with myself, but I was sure I had not. I moved the furniture from the door and quickly picked up my pistol. I was afraid to see the bedroom but knew I had to proceed and evaluate the whole situation.

I slowly opened the door. The raccoon that I had trapped was gone! But there was evidence he had been there. The pillow was on the floor, but the yellow trash can was still stuck beside the air conditioner. I went on to inspect the kitchen. When I found the empty chip bag any hopes of this being a dream were erased.

I called my brother, Bill, and told him I had a chore for him. I told him the horror story of my night. I did not hear much sympathy in his voice when he said "girl you are crazier than I thought.

Don't you know them suckers are dangerous, especially when they're hungry?"

"I hadn't stopped to think about that when I was looking that crazy raccoon in the eyes," I said a little upset. "All I wanted was him gone," I continued. "Can you come over and help me make sure that doesn't happen again?"

"Sure I will sis. I'll be over in a few minutes," he said with sweetness in his voice. I know by now he was smiling. He brought two pieces of paneling along with his hammer and nails. He nailed panel on each side of the air conditioner. He chuckled as he gave the last nail a final whack and said "If he gets in again he'll have to bring his own little hand-saw." We both sat and laughed.

"Great!" I let out a big sigh and said, "I trust that is the last of my night surprises. While you are here we might as well sit down and catch up on the latest news while we drink our coffee." We sat, talked and laughed the morning away.

Chapter 5

Later that day it was great to be able to sit and talk to my cousin Maureen. We laughed as we shared stories. My face became sober as I recalled my experience from the night before. She told me you have to be really careful and not cross them because they can be very dangerous. Then she told me how her pregnant pet raccoon had left the house a few days before and went into the woods. Even though they are pets, they will still go into the woods to have their babies. With a smile on my face I said, "Maybe it was your pet, she probably thought sense we are cousins it would be fine to come in and just help herself to a little late night snack". We both laughed at the thought.

The weekend ended much too quick. With the window down and the air blowing in my hair I could only think in spite of the unwelcomed visitor during the night, it turned out to be a terrific time with family and much needed rest. A great weekend.

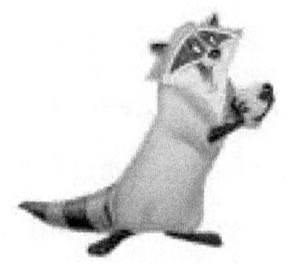

We don't know how much time we have on earth. It can be taken away in a blink of an eye.

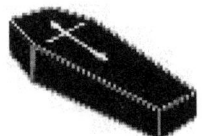

We need to always be ready to meet our maker. God does not tell us the day or time of our leaving this world.

IN A BLINK OF AN EYE

Chapter 1

He was dead!! I could see it but my mind refused to believe it. My hands shook with rage, my eyes smarted with tears as I tried not to let them flow down my cheeks. I reached over to close his lifeless eyes. I noticed he had beautiful blue eyes, ones he would never be able to open again. I was preparing his body for the awful things they would do in the morgue. They will split his chest open. Boy they will find the cause of death with no need to look further, but they will examine his brain anyway. I began to wonder why the first thing they tell you to do is "close the eyes" when a person dies. My best guess is so they don't look back at all those curiosity seekers that gawk and make asinine remarks like "Don't they look natural?" I felt rage filling me at the thought. "Of course they don't look natural! They are dead," I screamed inside myself. It would serve those curiosity seekers right if one time, while gawking during the viewing, one eye of the person would pop open. I am sure that would scare the pee right out of them. Then what would they say? I laughed to myself as I pictured such a thing. As for me, my casket is going to be closed and stay that way. If anyone dares open it I hope the Lord would grant me one last request. I would love to sit up and spit right in their eye. Then lay back down with a smile on my face. Maybe I could have something rigged up so water would squirt if the lid opened. Wouldn't that be a hoot? Oh well, this poor guy probably didn't share my views regarding the barbaric ways funerals are conducted anyway.

    I finished removing the tubes, needles, probes, and other paraphernalia attached to his body. He didn't need them now, and they hadn't helped him anyway. I couldn't help but notice his beautiful anatomy. His broad shoulders, flat belly and suntan lines made me think of an achiever, possibly a "Type A Personality" I thought. You know the kind, the ones that are real easy on the eyes. What an awful way to go. But had the ulcer not taken him I know by all signs a heart attack would. None the less what a senseless, useless waste! A life ended way too early.

Chapter 2

Stopping in my tracks I began to think of the events leading up to that very moment. The resident called me at 1:00 that afternoon and told me they were sitting on a G.I. bleeder. That meant they were to stabilize and control the hemorrhage. This could take any length of time. If they were successful the surgery could be done at another time after proper preparation. If not, the patient's condition would deteriorate and surgery would be imminent and swift. I did what I could to prepare for that event. I wrote his name on the schedule and noted that he was on the private wing of the Godhouse. His attending physician was the prominent in Jack-town and had been the first to receive a document from the American College of Surgeons attesting to his skills. I had thought "well, he is in good hands in case something did happen." Little did I know the end result would be what I face this very moment. Quickly my mind jumped back into the rest of the events that brought us to this point. I remember I stopped thinking about the doctor I had things to do. I knew I had to get a room empty, and find a table to put the patient on. This lasted well past quitting time and there were already two emergencies scheduled. Well, everybody will have to work overtime and both call teams will have to stay. Damn, I had forgotten Martha! Martha was a very special scrub nurse that stood 6 feet tall. Since I was the head nurse I put her on all the difficult cases. She was a gem to have around for emergencies. She could set up a case in ways no one else could, she never got flustered, no matter what. How fortunate we are to have her around. How could I have done this? Martha had been scrubbed since early and had sent me word by the "circulator" that her cycle had started. She needed to be relieved.

    I rushed over to the room where Martha was finally closing and everything seemed okay. "I'm so sorry Martha," I whispered. "Aw, that's all right. It has already run down my legs now, but nobody knows whether its mine or the bleeder that got lose," Martha quipped, pointing to the patient on the table. What a sense of humor she had. "Don't worry about it, I know you would have relieved me if you could have," she said. "Mother of Mary, what a team," I breathed. They were the glue that kept this macabre game of life and death together.

Chapter 3

The cases ended one by one, the rooms cleared, cleaned, and made ready for the next scene in the play of our OR. The call came. The bleeder had bled out. I was in my tenth hour of duty but yet another jolt of adrenaline sent me scurrying to set the stage for the bloody battle which we were surely to encounter. The unfortunates bled from the mouth, stomach, and the rectum. Oh, the smell, a cross between rotting fish and decaying flesh. They were all the same. You could smell them before you saw them. The doors opened, and in came the entourage of four people, two pumping blood, one pushing and another pulling the bed. Man, this was a bad one. He was brought in on a bed he was too sick to even move to a stretcher. I got my assistant to lay out the menagerie of instruments, supplies needed for the case. Prominent Cutting-Stitcher appeared along with the private Poison-Passer. "Crap," I thought, "this Poison-Passer is for the birds." I'll have my work cut out for me helping him. Besides being incompetent and slow as hell, he is a smart-ass. I never liked working with him and watched his every move. The patient was moved on to the cutting-stitching table. Patient had an I.V. line in his arm and another in his foot. Blood was being pumped through both and his pressure was holding. He also had a tube down his nose to the stomach, attached to suction, attempting in vain, to pull out the blood that clotted as soon as it hit his gastric juice. The Poison-Passer was lollygagging around foot line attaching syringes, probes, monitors, thither and yond. "He is going to be injecting the poison into his foot line!" I screamed inside just at the thought. That means nobody is going to be at the patient's head when the poison hits. When this is done it always causes the gastric muscle to contract causing anything in the stomach to eject through the mouth. "He'll drown," I panicked. I've got to stop this. "Let me inject him for you," I quickly said in a state of complete panic. "That way you can stay at the head of the table."

"You tend to your business, let me tend to mine" Poison-Passer said in a sarcastic manner.

I rapidly raced to the patient's head and grabbed the suction. I know someone needed to be there ready for what came next. It happened, the poison hit, the muscles contracted, blood gushed from the poor devil's mouth and nose. I suctioned frantically. The prominent stitcher and his helper had been scrubbing at the sink just outside. "We're in trouble," I yelled at the top of my lungs. I wanted everyone to know the severity of trouble we were encountering. They came rushing into the room, water dripping from their hands and arms. They JUST STOOD THERE WITH BLANK STARES ON THEIR FACES!!!!

The Poison-Passer and I worked desperately to clear the throat but the blood just kept coming. It was impossible to get an airway in to stop the blood from going to the lungs. John Doe literally drowned in his own blood. Then everyone left me to prepare him for his lonely journey to the morgue.

Chapter 4

"Yes, we have lost some," I leaned over and whispered to John Doe "but you shouldn't have been one of them, at least not like this. Not this time. You still had some good years left in you." Then I wiped the last smudge of blood from his lips, to finish getting him ready for his journey to the morgue. I forgot his real name that was on his chart from earlier. I had always tried not to attach names to the case procedures that passed through my hands. That way when questions were asked I could honestly say "I don't remember." I was going to try especially hard on this one because I never want to relate any part to anyone about what had happened this night. It was all like a horrible nightmare. I know that this scene will play, again and again in my mind's eyes, always.

The orderlies came and put his lifeless body on the stretcher to wheel him off to his final destination in our Godhouse. I stood and watched the orderlies accompany John Doe to the morgue as tears rolled down my cheeks. I prayed that God would comfort his family in this great loss.

"Now time to go home," I said as I wiped my brow. What a day!!!! In a blink of an eye a life lost, I thought, as I walked to my car shaking my head for the long drive home.

Someday a loving Hand will be laid upon our shoulder and this brief message will be given: "Come home."

Billy Graham

Conclusion

These stories are just a few atrocities that I have witnessed during my fifty years in the Health Care Industry. I felt they must be told because health care is apparently getting worse, instead of better. We have new challenges like MERSA and HIV. MERSA also is called the super bug. It was first labeled "hospital acquired" because that is where people got it. But so many patients unknowingly have been sent home with the infection, to the point that it is now called "Community Acquired." I thought I would share a little about MERSA it is a type of bacteria that is resistant to several types of antibiotics. These antibiotics are also used to treat other types of infections. These gems are continuously exposed to all types of antibiotics, therefore rendering them resistant.

Basic common sense rules are not followed like proper hand washing. Correct floor care, like changing the mop after each room, moping with the same water from one room to the other just carries the germs right along. There has been research done to find the source of germs. One hospital that was running test went so far as to culture physicians' neck ties. They found "bugs," but missed the obvious which came from the stethoscope hanging around their neck which they use from one patient to the next. I would suggest that you ask them to wipe it off with a sanitizer before they use it on you. Everyone's hygiene practice is important and crucial to your health.

Users beware, be diligent when being exposed to this necessary fearful industry. **Ask for Gods' guidance and direction when choosing a heath care provider and facility. Again I say as Paul does in I Thessalonians 5:17 "Pray without ceasing."**

www.ingramcontent.com/pod-product-compliance
Lightning Source LLC
Chambersburg PA
CBHW051203170526
45158CB00013B/120